The Transition Diet

The Transition Diet

**HOW TO TRANSITION TO A VEGETARIAN
OR SEMI-VEGETARIAN DIET**

David Yager

This book is dedicated to the liberation
of all beings from pain and suffering
"When our lives were touched by the True and Good Spiritual God
we changed our minds obsession and occupation with transitory
earthly matters and began to remember our Divine Origin"

Acknowledgments

With all my heart I express my love and gratitude to everyone who has supported me in the birth of this book. To my parents who inspired and supported me in seeking higher education and living at my highest potential. To my grandfather Frank who was a true American hero and an air mail pioneer. To Johnny for opening up a whole new world of Spirituality and the relation that diet and our way of life have in opening our hearts and minds. To Mary who constantly inspired me to keep going and get it done no matter what. To Susan for always supporting me with this book and in living a more independent and prosperous life. To my aunts, uncles and cousins for listening and sometimes acting on my "unasked for" diet and health lectures. To Diego who revived interest in Arnold Ehret's mucusless diet. To Daniel for patiently explaining to me aspects of the diet that never occurred to me. To Mark who inspired me to become a vegetarian and study spirituality. To Kevin who inspired me by becoming a University professor. To Fred who urged me to strive for excellence in everything. To Barbie who inspired me to excel in academics and not just athletics. To my football coaches Forrest, Mel and Gordy who pushed me beyond my self-made limitations. To Karen my junior college nutrition teacher who opened up the world of nutrition to me and inspired me to pursue it as a career. To Dr. Stern at U.C. Davis for allowing me to work on her research projects in obesity. To Dr. Ross and Dr. Radlefinger who opened up the world of social psychology and health education to me. Thank you India, and Tibet, and Japan, and China for teaching me holistic health and Eastern Wisdom. Thank you Ecuador for your climate and abundant fruits. Thank you Beatles for turning me on to Love and Spirituality in the sixties and to all musicians for your songs. Thank you Hollywood for your life changing movies like: Avatar, The Wizard of Oz, It's a Wonderful Life, Star Wars, The Lord of the Rings, Brother Sun, Sister Moon, A Field of Dreams, Little Buddha et al and for the Academy Awards show. Thank you NFL, NBA and MLB for all your wonderful and exciting games and inspiring me to excel in sports and in life. Thank you Oprah, Larry, Ellen, Mike, Merv and Johnny Carson. And above all, with all my heart, thank You Divine Father, Mother and Son for making it all possible.

CONTENTS

HOW TO DO THE TRANSITION DIET:
THE BASIC PRINCIPLES

THE TRANSITION DIET:
WHAT TO EAT AND HOW TO EAT IT

MINERALS, VITAMINS AND ESSENTIAL FATS

SUPPLEMENTS

HOW DIET AND STRESS AFFECTS OUR EMOTIONAL WELL-BEING

NATURAL LIVING, ITS ORIGIN AND RELATION TO OUR HEALTH

THE HEALING POWER OF EXERCISE

INTRODUCTION

TRANSITION TO A HEALTHY LIFE

Health is wealth. Health is our most important asset because without it all the love from others you could receive or all the money you could spend would be worthless. If you suffer constantly from a disease, you can't appreciate the love of others because you are too sick to receive their love. What good is money when you're in so much pain that nothing is enjoyable?

Health is beauty. When you see a beautiful woman or a handsome man, it means that they are healthy human beings who know how to live. We were not made to suffer quietly in sickness. The health laws of God and Nature need to be discovered, studied and practiced because ignorance of the law does not free us from punishment in the form of disease.

The English word health comes from the Old English word hale which means whole. To be healthy is to be whole and full of life. Holiness or whollyness is really health in mind, body, spirit and planet. To be spiritually enlightened is to be healthy and to live a natural, healthy lifestyle among the trees and plants and animals and bees, to commune with Nature and God and the planets. As it was in the beginning, so it is now and forever.

We've been wandering so long in the wilderness of an unhealthy, artificial way of life, struggling and suffering in the dark. We're sick and tired and just want to go home to paradise, our oasis in the desert of civilization. We've been there, done that, i.e. the industrialized, city thing, so now we're coming back full circle to our roots. It's what we're coming home to. We begin to realize that the most sophisticated and technologically advanced way of life is the simple purity of living a natural lifestyle, close to Nature.

This book is about transitioning to a healthier diet and lifestyle. Some people will be content to eat more fresh fruits, vegetables and cultured milk and less meat, white sugar, white flour, trans fats and junk foods. Those who "go the distance" and adopt a lacto-vegetarian diet high in fresh fruits and vegetables will reap more health benefits.

Elmer Verner (E. V.) McCollum, the discoverer of Vitamins A, B and D wrote, "I will only say that the lacto-vegetarian diet is a highly satisfactory regimen, if the food is properly selected. Meat eating is entirely unnecessary and indulgence in it is due to its palatability."

The French have the lowest heart disease of any nation in the world, according to 2009 UN/WHO figures, even lower than the Japanese and their diet is high in whole fat cheese, cream, butter and yogurt. French women eat one or two yogurts a day according to Mireille Guilliano, author of French Women Don't Get Fat. And the cheeses, General de Gaulle once quipped "How can you govern a country that has 246 varieties of cheese?"

The French don't have all the low-carb, low-fat, high-protein diet confusion or the latest nutrient supplement fad, just everyday whole foods; fresh local produce, French bread, wine, small portions of meat, plus butter, cream, yogurt and many varieties of whole fat cheeses.

The New York Times reporting on French life expectancy in 1911 wrote, "At the beginning of the last century (1800), the average duration barely exceeded the age of 30. In 1880 it was up to 40, and now varies between 47 and 48."

Now, just over 100 years later, life expectancy in France has sky-rocketed up. 2010 U.N. figures for life expectancy shows that France now averages 80.95 and the 2011 CIA World Factbook give France an average of 81.50.

But that is just the average. The Paris-based National Statistics Institute showed 20,106 centenarians as of January 1, 2013. Offset against a total population number of around 65 million, France's centenarian ratio is second only to Japan.

Frenchwoman Jeanne Calment lived to the age of 122 and is the oldest verified human in modern history. She was still riding a bicycle when she reached her 100th birthday.

The people of Monaco live the longest of any country in the world according to the CIA WORLD FACTBOOK 2012 edition. Men in Monaco live to be 85.74 and women live to be 93.77 and the average is 89.68. Monaco is completely surrounded by France and speaks French as its main language. Its ideal climate and high degree of wealth, plus the diet and lifestyle of the French all combine to make Monaco the longest living country on earth.

France and Monaco have semi-lacto-vegetarian diets since, for the most part, they eat small, controlled portions of meat and plenty of whole fat, grass-fed, dairy products.

Dan Buettner partnered with National Geographic and the National Institute on Aging and found pockets of longevity within certain countries. In Okinawa, Japan, Buettner found the longest disability-free life expectancy. Pork and fish are primarily eaten only on holidays but their everyday diet is mostly vegetables.

In Loma Linda, California, (23,261 pop. 2010) Seventh Day Adventists have a life expectancy that's 9 to 11 years greater than other Americans. About 50% of Seventh Day Adventists are lacto-ovo-vegetarians.

The mountain inhabitants in Sardinia, Italy, have the highest number of male centenarians in the world (10.8 per 1,000 newborns). In the isolated mountain villages of Sardinia they only eat pork or lamb on special occasions and only a little, but on a daily basis they eat plenty of cheese, especially pecorino cheese made from sheep's milk. Their very low meat consumption and high vegetable and cheese consumption makes them virtually lacto-vegetarians.

VEGETARIANS HAVE LESS DISEASE AND LIVE LONGER

Research from Harvard suggests even moderate consumption of red meat, as little as one serving a day, poses a more serious health risk than first thought (Pan et al., 2012). Frank Hu, a professor of nutrition and epidemiology at Harvard says, "This study provides clear evidence that regular consumption of red meat, especially processed meat, contributes substantially to premature death."

The Adventist Mortality Study (1960–1965) showed that Adventist men lived 6.2 years longer than non-Adventist men in the concurrent American Cancer Society Study and Adventist women had a 3.7-year advantage over their counterparts. It consisted of 22,940 California Adventists and entailed an intensive 5-year follow-up and a more informal 25-year follow-up. The statistics were based on life table analyses. About 50 percent were lacto-ovo-vegetarians. Comparing death rates of Adventists compared to other Californians:

66% lower Coronary heart disease for Adventist men
98% lower Coronary heart disease for Adventist women
60% lower death rate from all cancers for Adventist men
76% lower death rate from all cancers for Adventist women

21% lower Lung cancer
62% lower Colorectal cancer
85% lower Breast cancer

The Adventist Health Study 1 or (AHS-1) from 1974–1988 involved approximately 34,000 Californian Adventists over 25 years of age. Unlike the mortality study, the purpose was to find out which components of the Adventist lifestyle give protection against disease. The data has been studied for more than a decade and the findings link diet to cancer and coronary heart disease.

Of the 34,192 participants, all members of the Seventh-day Adventist church: 29 percent were vegetarian, while 7-10 percent of the vegetarians were vegan. Compared to non-vegetarians the above vegetarians had about:

1/2 the high blood pressure and diabetes
1/2 the colon cancer
2/3 the rheumatoid arthritis and prostate cancer
Breast, lung, & uterine cancers tended to be lower in vegetarians but could have been due to random chance. The data has been studied for more than a decade and the findings link diet to cancer and coronary heart disease.

Two important things that this study found are: 1. Adventist men live 7.3 years longer and Adventist women live 4.4 years longer than other Californians on average and 2. Increasing consumption of red and white meat was associated with an increase of colon cancer.

THE TRANSITION DIET

TRANSITION: 1. a: passage from one state, stage, subject, or place to another: CHANGE. b: an evolution from one stage, or style to another. Merriam-Webster Dictionary

The Transition Diet is a systematic method to help you transition gracefully to a lacto-vegetarian or semi-lacto-vegetarian diet. In order to achieve radiant health a gentle and long term house-cleaning of your body is required. Disease, in most cases, is the result of eating improper, unnatural, processed foods or in other words; malnutrition. It is also due to internal toxicity due to wrong or chemically contaminated food and environmental pollution. Excess stress, birth defects and genetics also play a part.

The body's inherent wisdom is always working to heal wounds and maintain a steady state, free of toxic matter like during a cold when copious amounts of mucus are expelled. The rate of waste material and mucus being eliminated naturally by the body can be artfully controlled by the diet.

Heavier, mucus forming foods like cooked grains, potatoes, mayonnaise, olive oil and lighter, steamed, mucusless starchy vegetables are used to slow down the rate of elimination. This is important because a slower elimination rate uses less of the body's vital energy to detoxify itself.

Transitioning too quickly only depletes one's vital energy reserves. There are general principles of the transition system that can be applied to everyone, with minor variations, thus allowing a transition with a minimum of suffering.

Virtually everyone has been eating an unhealthy diet since childhood, a diet of pasteurized milk, fried eggs, bacon, hot dogs, cheeseburgers, steak, French fries, white bread, donuts, candy, ice cream, candy and pesticide laden fruits and vegetables.

When someone skips a meal or doesn't eat for a whole day the excess mucus and toxic material stored in the cellular spaces and intestine floods into the bloodstream making them ill. Even vegetarians or vegans can get toxicity symptoms from the toxic material being released too quickly from their cells, from 15, 20 or even 30 or more years of eating a highly toxic conventional diet.

When your nose is stuffed up or your throat is full of phlegm it means you have an excess of mucus. If your sinuses are not plugged up your voice really resonates in a beautiful tone. People can look pasty white and bloated due to eating too many mucus forming foods.

Each person is more or less congested with mucus and toxic waste products depending on their past eating habits and life-style and thus has to modify the basic transition plan to their specific needs.

A gradual and slow change from an ordinary, omnivorous, (meat, potatoes, rice, bread, dairy, fruits, vegetables) diet to a natural, vegetarian diet is needed to avoid shocking the body. Changing your diet requires patience and a gentleness that doesn't force things.

The idea of a gradual transition from a regular omnivorous diet to a natural diet we owe in part to Arnold Ehret and the many people in Spain, the United Kingdom and the United States who have revived, clarified and added personal insights to his work to create a new and updated, modern day transition diet. This diet has been proven effective by many case studies in Spain, the United Kingdom and the United States.

TRANSITION TO
HEALTH AND WHOLENESS

The word health means to be whole or bodily sound. The word health also comes from Helios the Greek Sun God represented by Apollo. The sun is the source of the whole of life. Holy is another word for a whole or healthy person. Wholeness and (w)holistic means that the body, mind and spirit are working as a harmonious whole.

To feel great you've got to be healthy. To have mental and spiritual health one needs bodily health. Bodily health depends mostly on what you eat and drink. It's that simple, you're not going to be a great, loving, happy person if you're not feeding your body right.

Euphoria is what we want, feeling great! Everybody talks about a natural high but nobody tells you what to eat. Eating organic, tree-ripened fruit gets you high and not an artificial high like on drugs. Fresh, ripe to perfection figs can do it, as can mangos, peaches, apples, or any high quality fruit.

But don't get hooked and think you can live on just fruit and feel exuberant all the time because first you need to do a slow and gradual transition to prepare your toxic body for its ideal foods. Vegetables and fruits, high in living, bioactive water (full of vitamins, enzymes and organic minerals) plus cultured milk products like cheese and yogurt are our ideal foods. Health authorities agree that fruits and vegetables are the healthiest of foods. The ancient science of yoga states that fruit is the most sattvic or spiritual and highest food.

There are literally thousands of varieties of fruits and vegetables (mangos, strawberries, apples, tomatoes, cucumbers, lettuce, spinach, kale etc.) to choose from. Many fail to thrive on a natural fruit, vegetable and cultured milk based diet because they don't detoxify their body first using a systematic and lengthy transition and they eat too many fruits and not enough vegetables and cultured milk products.

They feel great for a few weeks or months on just fruit or just fruit and vegetables, then wham, they feel horrible, weak, jittery and they binge-out on their old favorite cooked dishes, pizza or a few whole avocados. These foods are so heavy they get sick with a sore throat, earache and indigestion. Understanding the principles of dietary transition, you would have known to eat a big, green, leafy salad dressed with fat and protein, cooked starchy vegetables like broccoli and cooked brown rice (whole grain) or potatoes.

Vegetables, fruits, tender greens, grasses, herbs and cultured milk are the ideal foods of humans but only after a thorough purification. The missing key that has held people back for so long unable to find the way back to ideal health, has been a systematic, gradual transition that allows the body to slowly adapt to a new diet and way of life.

This gradual, dietary transition has finally been re-discovered thanks to the work of various teachers and students of natural living. We have been given a wonderful opportunity to heal ourselves through diet and lifestyle changes. The purpose of this book is to explain this revolutionary diet and lifestyle transition, so that you can achieve for yourself optimum or "paradise" health and happiness.

TRANSITION TO OUR NATURAL DIET

Ok we are toxic and mucus congested, you may be asking, but how did we get this way? What is it that we eat that is causing the problem? What diet do we transition to? What is our natural diet, the eating of which will give us natural health? We can look to many sources for the answer to these questions; biology, physiology, medical research, anthropology, the bible, historians and the great writers and scientists who have adopted a vegetarian diet such as Benjamin Franklin, Albert Einstein, Linus Pauling, Leonardo Da Vinci, Thomas Edison, Mahatma Ghandi, John Wesley (founder of the Methodists), Clement of Alexandria, Jerome, Tertullian, John Chrysostom, Origen, Ellen G. White, Albert Schweitzer, Sylvester Graham (Graham crackers), Dr. John H. Kellogg (famous health resort director, his brother invented corn flakes) and Leo Tolstoy.

THE NATURAL DIET OF HUMANS

Charles Darwin, the well known author of the theory of evolution, in his book *The Descent of Man* (1871), writes, "Although we know nothing for certain about the time or place that man shed the thick hair that covered him, with much probability of being right we could say that he must have lived in a warm country where conditions were favourable to the frugivorous way of life which, to judge from analogies, must have been the way man lived."

Dr. Alan Walker (1996) in his book *The Wisdom of the Bones* states, "The microwear studies suggested a largely frugivorous (fruit based with tender vegetation, which don't scar the teeth) diet for the robust australopithecines from East and South Africa, while South African gracile australopithecines had a vegetarian but less course and abrasive diet" (p. 168).

Australopithecines is a genus which first occurred 4 million years ago and became extinct 2 million years ago after evolving into the Homo genus (Homo habilis, Homo sapiens sapiens etc.). After examining Homo erectus "1808" Dr. Walker found evidence of meat eating in the enamel wear and stated, "Hominids had made an important dietary transition from a more plant-based to a more animal-based diet, a change that must have occurred later than Australopithecus and Paranthropus."

Subsequent research in the late 1980s revealed that Australopithecus also included small amounts of flesh, seeds and vegetable foods and that the species that followed, Homo habilis, included significant amounts of meat in their diet of mostly fruits and vegetables.

4

Our distant relatives began eating mostly fruit and tender vegetation supplemented by seeds and small amounts of meat and then later began eating large amounts of meat. This was the beginning of the Paleolithic or Stone Age hunter gatherer diet (about 2,500,000 to 10,000-8,500 years ago) of wild game, fruit, vegetables, nuts and seeds. Some 10,000, or possibly even 15,000 years ago, man began cultivating and eating a lot of grains during the Neolithic or New Stone Age period.

The Paleo or hunter gatherer diet is healthier than a Neolithic cooked grain based diet (due to the phytic acid and anti-nutrients), however a lacto-vegetarian diet based on fruits and vegetables is even healthier, because it returns us closer to the original, natural diet of mankind which was high in fruit and vegetation and low in meat and seed consumption. As a protein source grass-fed dairy products are healthier than meat (increased mortality) and seeds (phytic acid demineralization, reactive polyunsaturated fats and anti-nutrients). We are vegetarians or more specifically frugivores by design, who eat fruit, vegetables and a protein and fat source. As a protein and fat source grass-fed dairy is healthier than meat, fish, nuts and seeds.

We have already seen how meat is an unhealthy according to the studies cited previously, now we will see why nuts and seeds are also unhealthy.

Nuts and seeds are the reproductive vehicle of the plant. Some animals, like birds and squirrels, are adapted to eating them. The gizzard is a bird's specialized digestive system which helps it digest coarse seeds.

Humans are not birds nor rodents nor animals, they are human, even though Darwin classified them as animals. They are a higher form of being, a spiritually and mentally more advanced life form than animals and therefore they require a food that supports their advanced spiritual and intellectual capacity. Linus Pauling, the double Noble prize laureate, has pointed out that fruit best facilitates the neurotransmitters of the brain due to their high vitamin C content. Vegetables have low concentrations of vitamin C and the other food groups have very little.

Nuts and seeds are low in living water content and very high in fat and protein which is the opposite of mother's milk, the first food of humans, which is very low in protein and fat and high in living water. Living water is water that has been activated by a living plant, human or animal, with living enzymes, vitamins and organic minerals. Dead earth water or rain water has not been activated with these living elements. Fruit and vegetables are naturally high in living water and low in protein and fat which is similar to mother's milk.

Nuts are high in polyunsaturated fats which are known to be cancer and heart disease causing. Nature designed the seed to contain lots of polyunsaturated oil so that if an animal ate it, it would get indigestion and therefore avoid it in the future. Nuts and seeds are mucus forming because the body must produce extra mucus in order to protect itself from the toxic nature of the substances they contain.

The purpose of a nut or seed is to reproduce its kind as it states in Genesis of the Bible. Birds and other animals do eat them but they are adapted to do so. Humans are meant to care for and propagate fruit trees and vegetable plants throughout creation by saving the seed and planting it. The trees and plants in turn provide living water, enzymes, organic minerals and vitamins for our sustenance. This is the natural, symbiotic relationship between humans, fruit trees and vegetable plants. In addition humans care for grazing animals like cows, sheep, goats, buffalo and camels and in turn they provide milk.

Another reason nuts, seeds and grains are unhealthy is due to their phytic acid content, a substance that can block mineral absorption.

PHYTIC ACID CAN BLOCK
MINERAL ABSORPTION

Phytate intake in the U.S. and the U.K. on average ranges between 631 and 746 mg per day; the average in Finland is 370 mg; in Italy it is 219 mg; and in Sweden a mere 180 mg per day. In the context of a diet rich in calcium, vitamin D, vitamin A, vitamin C, good fats and lacto-fermented foods, most people will do fine on an estimated 400-800 mg per day. Over 800 mg phytic acid per day is not recommended. For those suffering from tooth decay, bone loss or mineral deficiencies, a phytate intake of 150-400 mg would be advised. For children under age six, pregnant women or those with serious illnesses, it is best to consume a diet as low in phytic acid as possible.

Phytic Acid Content of Foods, mg/gm approximate
White bread 1.48
Oat bread 5.16

Bran bread 7.53
Soy bread 5.51
Mixed-grains bread 3.81
Whole wheat bread 4.74
Source: Phytic acid content in milled cereal products and breads, Rosa Ma Garcia-Estepa, Eduardo Guerra-Hernandez, Belen Garcia-Villanova, Food Research International 32 (1999) 217-221.

The average piece of bread is one ounce or 28 grams. One slice of whole wheat bread contains about 133 mg phytate, if you ate 4 slices per day that would be 531 mg. One slice of white bread has about 41 mg phytic acid, if you ate 4 slices that would be about 166 mg. For healing tooth decay and preventing it, white bread, French bread and sourdough rye or buckwheat bread are the best ways to keep your phytic acid intact to a minimum.

PHYTATES, As Percentage of Weight
Cornbread 1.36
Whole wheat bread 0.43-1.05
Wheat bran muffin 0.77-1.27
Popped corn 0.6
Rye 0.41
Pumpernickel 0.16
White bread 0.03-.23
French bread 0.03
Sourdough rye 0.03
Soured buckwheat 0.03
Sesame, dehulled 5.36
Almond 1.14
Walnut 0.98
Peanut 0.82
Peanut Roasted 0.95
Peanut Sprouted 0.61
Brazil Nut 1.72
Source: Reddy NR and others. Food Phytates, 1st edition, CRC Press, 2001, pages 30-32

Nuts contain about the same level of phytic acid as grains says Ramiel Nagel in, *Are Grains the Hidden Reason for many Modern Diseases including Tooth Cavities?* (http://www.healingourchildren.org/whole-grains-pregnancy). He goes on to say, "Both Edward and May Mellanby's decades of research show that oatmeal interferes more than any other grain studied with tooth mineralization. Intermediate interference of tooth mineralization occurs from corn, rye, barley and rice. Wheat germ, corn germ and other grain germs have a 'baneful' effect on teeth.

White flour interferes the least with tooth mineralization. That white flour does not interfere as much with tooth mineralization corresponds with Weston Price's feeding experiments discussed in chapter two in which cavity-ridden school children consumed two meals per day consisting of white flour, and one excellent meal per day with nutrient-dense foods. Even while consuming the white flour the children all became immune to tooth cavities.

Sprouting only removes between 20-30% of phytic acid after two or three days for beans, seeds, and grains under laboratory conditions at a constant 77 degrees Fahrenheit. Yeasted breads have 40-80% of their phytic acid intact in their finished product. If a yeasted bread is made with unbleached white flour, however, it will not have much phytic acid (white bread 0.03-.23% by weight). Another deadly food for teeth is commercially made sprouted grain products from whole grains."

"If you have severe tooth cavities, or have some nagging cavities that do not heal, consider avoiding nuts entirely until the problem resolves. Be careful with almonds; they seem to be very high in plant toxins. The skins must be removed.

I think nuts are delicious—especially when they have been sprouted and low-temperature dehydrated, and then roasted to eliminate a large amount of phytic acid. It seems almost universal that indigenous cultures cooked their nuts in some way, such as adding them to meat soups and stews. The problem people have with nuts is that they are consuming too many raw, which means they are high in phytic acid, and too much as a staple, rather than as a part of a wholesome diet."

Roasted peanuts have a very high phytic acid content (0.95 as Percentage of Weight), so just cooking them has little effect in reducing phytic acid. Sprouting peanuts does reduce the phytic acid but still they are high at 0.61. It is best to leave nuts alone because later we will see that they are too high in phosphorus which will also prevent calcium from being assimilated.

We've been led to believe that whole grain wheat bread is better than white bread, yet white bread has practically no phytic acid to interfere with the absorption of calcium and other minerals. As a kid growing up in the 60's in America we always had white bread sandwiches, but we also ate butter, eggs, whole milk, whole cheese and mayonnaise which are high in vitamin D, K and calcium which help maintain strong teeth.

It wasn't until the early 70's that whole wheat bread and oat based granola, both high in mineral blocking phytates, were forced on the American public by the new hippie, back to nature movement. At the same time butter and whole milk were being touted as evil because their saturated fat and cholesterol were causing heart disease. Trans fat loaded and vitamin K deficient margarine was the healthy alternative, but in reality it was the cause of the problem.

So this double whammy, of excess phytic acid from whole grains and the loss of natural vitamin D and K found in butter and whole milk products, was what played havoc on our teeth and bones. Even though white flour has no phytic acid it still is highly mucus forming (colds, runny noses) and will form a sticky paste if mixed with water.

Even if you could get all the phytic acid out of nuts, seeds and beans, you would still have the problem of them having too much phosphorus.

GRAINS

"With the consuming of grains the degeneration of man began," holds anthropology Professor R. D. McCracken of the University of California. In 10,000 years of grain cultivation man has destroyed 90% of the forests from Spain to India in order to plant this crop. In the U.S. it took only 300 years. In the last 50 years or so, grain cultivation has been replaced by animal cultivation as a major cause of deforestation.

Mankind is smothering to death from a lack of oxygen in the air and an excess of carbon dioxide due to the cutting of the forests and fuel burning. This excess carbon dioxide also causes the greenhouse effect which destabilizes the global climate.

Grains produce bread the so called "Staff of Life" which has really destroyed mankind in body and environment. Grains mine the body of minerals and nutrients and likewise drain the soil of minerals and nutrients, until finally it can only support a desert-like environment. Grains contain phytates which bind minerals preventing their physiological assimilation. Anti-nutrients in cereal grains directly impair vitamin D metabolism which is crucial to calcium absorption (Batchelor 1983; Clement 1987).

Loren Cordain has shown in *The Late Role of Grains and Legumes in the Human Diet, and Biochemical Evidence of their Evolutionary Discordance* (1999) that high grain consumption (one that constitutes 50% or more of the diet) causes mineral (calcium and phosphorus) deficiency diseases such as bone softening (rickets in children and osteomalcea in adults) (Dagnelie 1990) and retarded skeletal growth due to lack of zinc (Golub 1996).

Chuang Tsu wrote about the "Spiritualized man" who "does not eat any of the 5 grains, but inhales the air and drinks the dew." The "five grains" (now more than five) are used worldwide including; wheat, rice, corn, rye, barley, millet, sorghum and oats, all of which can cause health problems.

Grains can cause a scaly, eczema-like skin condition in people who have detoxified their body through diet and fasting. Many people are allergic to gluten, a protein found in wheat, rye, barley, oats and spelt. Sprouted grain breads are offered as the alternative, yet they are still very high in phosphorus which can prevent mineral absorption.

BEANS

Are beans our natural diet? Pythagoras, the well known Greek mathematician, philosopher and founder of the vegetarian movement in the Western world, taught that beans are a forbidden food.

Modern science has proven him right showing that beans, which are legumes, are indigestible and toxic (Liener, 1994), (Gupta, 1987) and not even cooking can eliminate their toxic elements (Grant, 1982). Beans in their cooked form are infamous for causing gas which is caused by indigestible carbohydrates.

The soybean has a higher phytate content than any other grain or legume that has been studied. It seems to be highly resistant to many phytate reducing techniques such as long, slow cooking. Only a long period of fermentation will significantly reduce the phytate content of soybeans.

Fermented products such as tempeh, miso (too high in salt) and soy sauce (high in salt) are more easily digested, but the use of tofu, soy milk, soy meat and soy yogurt, high in phytates, is unhealthy. Vegetarians who consume tofu, soy milk, soy meat and soy yogurt as a substitute for meat and dairy products risk severe mineral deficiencies due to their high phytate content.

In the production of soy milk in order to remove as much of the trypsin inhibitor content as possible, the beans are first soaked in an alkaline solution. The pureed solution is then heated to about 115 degrees Centigrade in a pressure cooker. This method destroys most, but not all, of the anti-nutrients but unfortunately it has the side effect of denaturing the proteins so that they become very difficult to digest and much reduced in effectiveness.

The phytate content remains in soy milk to block the uptake of essential minerals like calcium, magnesium, iron and zinc. The alkaline soaking solution produces a carcinogen, lysinealine. Soy yogurt is made from soy milk and is therefore not as healthy as fermented soy foods.

Trypsin inhibitors in soy interfere with protein digestion and may cause pancreatic disorders. Soy phytoestrogens disrupt endocrine function and may cause infertility and breast cancer. Soy phytoestrogens cause hypothyroidism and may cause thyroid cancer. Infant soy formula has been linked to autoimmune thyroid disease.

In Okinawa, Japan, Dan Buettner, author of *The Blue Zones*, found the longest disability-free life expectancy. Sweet potatoes, bean sprouts, onions, and green peppers are prominent in the diet. Vegetables (sweet potato mostly), grains (75% less rice and noodles than the Japanese mainland), and fruits make up 72% of the diet by weight. Soy and seaweed provide another 14%. 6% of total caloric intake is in the form of soy and other legumes. Meat, poultry, and eggs account for just 3% of the diet, fish about 11%.

The emphasis is on dark green vegetables and seaweed rich in calcium. The Okinawans, like other Japanese, don't eat much dairy.

The Okinawan diet derives most of its calories from sweet potato. Tofu and soy sauce only constitute 6% of the total calories. In Japan fermented tofu is largely unknown but in Okinawa fermented tofu is well known. Fermented tofu has less phytic acid and trypsin inhibitors than unfermented tofu.

In 100 grams or about 3.5 ounces of nigari (hard type) tofu there is 5.6 grams of polyunsaturated fat; 4971 mg omega-6 and 667 mg omega-3. Tofu is a high polyunsaturated fat food compared to an equal 100 grams of mozzarella whole milk cheese with 0.8 grams polyunsaturated fat. Polyunsaturated fats can cause heart disease and hypothyroidism. I will cover this in detail later.

The fact that Okinawans enjoy a high degree of longevity and health is not because they consume soy, due to the fact it is eaten in small amounts (6% of total calories) compared to the staples of sweet potato, vegetables, seaweed and small amounts of fish and pork. The Okinawan diet does not justify the wholesale consumption of non-fermented soy foods like soy milk, soy yogurt, soy cheese, soy ice cream, soy nuts and unfermented tofu. Small amounts of fermented soy tempeh and fermented tofu if digestible would be ok, but miso and soy sauce are too high in blood pressure raising salt.

THE CALCIUM/PHOSPHORUS RATIO

If you eat foods that have more phosphorus than calcium, they will rob your teeth and bones of calcium because any excess phosphorus is excreted by the kidney along with calcium in the body.

There is a saying "as goes phosphorus, so goes calcium". What this means is that for every gram of phosphorus ingested in the diet, the body must match that with another gram of calcium before the phosphorus can be absorbed through the intestinal wall into the bloodstream. If the required calcium is not available from the diet, the body will obtain it from wherever it can, such as from the storage deposits in the teeth and bones.

Grains, beans, sprouts, nuts and seeds are all too high in phosphorus and too low in calcium and will thus drain your body of its calcium reserves stored in the teeth and bones.

"Your kidneys regulate how much phosphorus is in your blood. When phosphorus gets too high, your kidneys excrete the extra. Unfortunately, phosphorus and calcium are closely associated and calcium gets excreted along with the phosphorus.", says Joanne Larsen MS, RD, LD from the Ask the Dietitian website. Human milk has a calcium:phosphorus ratio of 2:1 so foods should be near this ratio because that is what our bodies first used as a food source.

Papaya is a fair calcium food. One cup of mashed papaya pulp has 55 mg calcium and only 12 mg phosphorus. 4 cups or one liter of papaya pulp has 172 net mgs of calcium; 220 mg calcium minus 48 mg phosphorus gives 172 mg calcium. Spinach is an excellent source of net calcium. Spinach has a Ca to P ratio of 2.02:1 giving 46 net grams of absorbable calcium.

Dr. Norman Walker, author of *Raw Vegetable Juices,* held that oxalic acid in its cooked form binds irreversibly with calcium and prevents its absorption. An excess of cooked oxalic acid may also form oxalic acid crystals in the kidney. Dr. Walker claimed oxalic acid stones and calcium blockage do not occur eating raw spinach because the organic oxalic acid can be metabolized appropriately. Oxalic acid in its raw form is one of the important nutrients needed to maintain tone and peristalsis of the bowel.

Dandelion greens contain 187 mg calcium and 66 mg phosphorus in every 100 grams giving it a net calcium yield of 121 mg. This is one of the of the highest calcium sources in the vegetable realm and it's a freely growing, widespread weed.

Sea vegetables are high in calcium, magnesium and potassium. Dulse has 567.0 mg calcium and 270.0 mg phosphorus per 100 grams yielding 297 mg calcium. Wakame or Alaria marginata has 1300.0 mg calcium and 260.0 mg phosphorus yielding 1040 mg calcium per 100 grams. Hijiki has 1,400.0 mg calcium per 100 grams and just 59 mg phosphorus yielding 1,341 mg calcium making it the highest source of calcium among sea vegetables. Flaked sea vegetables can be used as seasoners instead of salt. Maine Coast Sea Vegetables has many tasty sea vegetables and seasoners to choose from and they have been tested as both radiation and pollution free. Grass-fed, pasture-raised dairy products are good sources of calcium.

According to USDA (United States Department of Agriculture) figures broccoli has 40 mg of calcium and 67 mg phosphorus for each 100 gram serving giving a net loss of calcium of 27 mg. That would give broccoli 1 mg calcium for every 1.4 mg phosphorus so it would rob your body's calcium by .4 mg for every one mg phosphorus that is eaten. They probably used commercial produce grown on mineral deficient soil. Using organic broccoli probably would yield a higher calcium to phosphorus ratio.

Common white mushrooms may be the worst offenders in calcium theft. They contain, in 100 grams, 86 mgs phosphorus and only 3 mg calcium giving it a 1:28.7 Ca:P ratio. Each mg of phosphorus will rob one milligram of calcium from your teeth and bones. Just four large mushrooms (about 100 gm) will rob your body of about 83 mg of calcium.

Most people think that carrots are rich in calcium with 24 milligrams per 100 grams but they contain 42 mg phosphorus according to USDA figures. Again organic carrots may have a more balanced mineral content. According to USDA figures, which are used by nutritiondata.self.com, a cup of carrot juice will rob your body of about 42 mg of calcium and a quart will rob 168 mg of calcium from your body. One cup of carrot juice contains 56.6 mg of calcium and 99.1 mg of phosphorus according to nutritiondata.self.com.

Carrot juice should be mixed with spinach, celery, parsley and dandelion to balance any possible calcium deficit. Cucumber has a net negative calcium balance. In one large cucumber (about 300 gms) there are 48 mg calcium and 72 mg phosphorus giving a net drain of 24 mg of calcium. Yet, cucumber is high in silica and silica is converted to calcium by the body by biological transmutation, thus making up for its excess phosphorus. Silica is good for the skin, tendons and ligaments.

If the oxalic acid in vegetables like Swiss chard is a concern then use broccoli, cauliflower and cabbage which have no to low oxalate content. Swiss chard, spinach and other oxalate containing vegetables when cooked form an interlocking compound with calcium destroying its nourishing value. There are a few, relatively rare health conditions that require strict oxalate restriction. About 80% of kidney stones formed by adults in the U.S. are calcium oxalate stones. High refined sugar intake, high protein intake and high sodium intake contribute to stone formation. One study showed that in women who drank ½ to 1 liter of apple, grapefruit or orange juice daily, their urinary pH value and citric acid excretion increased, significantly dropping their risk of forming calcium oxalate stones.

Virginia Worthington, a clinical nutritionist with a doctorate in nutrition from Johns Hopkins, published a review (2001) of 41 studies comparing the nutritional value of organic and conventional produce. Dr. Worthington concluded that organic produce had on average 27 percent more vitamin C, 21.1 percent more iron, 29.3 percent more magnesium and 13.6 percent more phosphorous than conventional produce.

Charles Benbrook, chief scientist at the Organic Center and a former executive director of the Board on Agriculture of the National Academy of Sciences, found that in 85 percent of the comparable data points, produce from organic farms had higher levels of antioxidants than did produce from conventional farms. On average, antioxidant levels in organic produce were 30 percent higher. Therefore, to get more vitamins, minerals and antioxidants in your diet choose organic or naturally grown produce.

THE IMPORTANCE OF GRASS-FED DAIRY PRODUCTS

FULL FAT DAIRY PRODUCTS
ARE GOOD FOR YOU

Government agencies and the food industry have spent the last 30 years telling you to eat low-fat dairy when most studies are actually more consistent with the idea that dairy fat reduces the risk of heart disease.

A study of 1000 in Sweden found that people that consumed the most dairy fat were at lower risk of heart attack (Warensjö et al, 2010). For women, the risk was reduced by 26 percent, for men the risk was 9 percent lower.

A 2010 study showed that people who ate the most full-fat dairy had a 69% lower risk of cardiovascular death than those who ate the least (Bonthuis, Hughes, Ibiebele, Green, & van der Pols, 2010). The study lasted 16 years and used a sample of 1529 adult Australians aged 25–78 years. People who avoided dairy or consumed low-fat dairy had more than three times the risk of dying of coronary heart disease or stroke than people who ate the most full-fat diary.

A literature review of 10 studies found that milk drinking is associated with a small, but significant reduction in heart disease and stroke risk (Elwood, Pickering, Hughes, Fehily, & Ness, 2004)

The Rotterdam study of 4807 people found that high vitamin K2 intake was linked to a lower risk of fatal heart attack, aortic calcification and overall mortality (Geleijnse, 2004). Most of the vitamin K2 came from full-fat cheese.

The Caerphilly study (Elwood et al, 2005) used a representative population sample of men in South Wales, aged 45-59 between 1979-83 and followed them for 20 years. The results of the study showed that the subjects who drank more than the median amount of milk had a reduced risk of stroke, and possibly a reduced risk of heart attack.

T. Colin Campbell, author of *The China Study* linked isolated casein, a protein in dairy products, with cancer. He also believes that all animal proteins cause cancer and one should adopt a strict vegan diet. What Campbell neglected to observe is that whey, another protein found in dairy, has anti-cancer effects that completely cancel out the cancer-promoting effects of casein. This leads to the question; what if the butterfat and whey was tested with the casein as occurs naturally in dairy products? It would not cause tumors because it has already been proven that whey cancels out the cancer promoting qualities of casein. Another of Campbell's studies showed that tumor growth induced by animal protein could be inhibited by swapping the sources of fat in the diet (fish oil instead of corn oil). This leads to the question; what effect does butterfat and especially grass-fed butterfat have on the inhibition of tumor growth? All of this goes to show that whole foods must be studied and not isolated casein.

SATURATED FATS AND CHOLESTEROL DO NOT CAUSE HEART DISEASE

The French eat high cholesterol, high saturated fat whole milk cheeses, yogurt, cream, dressing, sauces and butter, yet they have the lowest rate of heart disease of any developed country according to World Health Organization (WHO) figures.

On the island of Kitava in Papua New Guinea the non-industrialized natives eat a diet that derives 21% of its calories from fat, 17% of which is saturated fat found in coconuts. Heart disease and stroke are absent or extremely rare on Kitava (Lindeberg & Lundh, 1993).

The myth that animal fat, as found in whole milk cheeses, yogurt and butter, cause heart disease all started with the K-ration in World War II which was named after Dr. Ancel Keys using the first letter of his last name. He developed a high calorie food package of dried meat, dried biscuits etc. which helped win the war and made Dr. Keys quite famous. During the Korean War in 1953 Army and Marine doctors shocked the world when they found that the young men they did autopsies on had plaque in their arteries, which was usually only seen in older men.

People in the United States were dying of heart disease in epidemic proportions. Dr. Ancel Keyes was well respected and came up in 1953 with the theory that cholesterol and saturated fat was the cause of heart disease and everyone, desperate for a cure, accepted it as fact due to the prestige he held. The problem is that at that time trans fats were classified as saturated fats, so foods made with them were classified as saturated fats and subsequent studies put the blame on saturated fats and not on trans and polyunsaturated fats which are the real killers.

Just 3 years later Ancel Keys changed his mind and said in 1956, "In the adult man the serum cholesterol level is essentially independent of the cholesterol intake over the whole range of human diets." And in 1997, "There's no connection whatsoever between cholesterol in food and cholesterol in blood. And we've known that all along. Cholesterol in the diet doesn't matter at all unless you happen to be a chicken or a rabbit." Ancel Keys, Ph.D., professor emeritus at the University of Minnesota 1997.

So, why aren't the major television networks, newspapers and magazines hammering home this point? Because it keeps the low-fat and non-fat food manufacturers, the statin drug makers and the margarine manufacturers in business.

There is more money to be made in promoting blood cholesterol lowering drugs, non-fat and low-fat dairy and other food products, margarine, chemically extracted oils and hydrogenated shortenings than telling the truth that natural, whole fat cheese, yogurt, cottage cheese, butter and coconut oil do not cause heart disease.

The hydrogenation process was discovered around the turn of the 20th century, making it possible to produce partially hydrogenated fat, often referred to as trans fatty acid or trans fat. This was the first man-made fat to join our food supply. Trans fats are produced in the process that adds hydrogen to liquid vegetable oils in order to make them into solids.

The first commercial product was Crisco introduced by Proctor and Gamble back in 1911. Cheap vegetable oil was heated at high temperature producing a solid fat imitating lard, shortening (a mixture of vegetable oil and pig fat or beef tallow) and butter. Hydrogenation was cheaper and easier than making shortening so the big food companies decided to use just vegetable oil and hydrogenate it.

Trans fat gained widespread popularity during World War II, when many people began using margarine and shortening as alternatives to rationed butter.

I remember growing up in the 1960s and using Crisco on everything like fried chicken, French fries and cakes.

The commercials for margarine were quite famous and popular like, "It's not nice to fool Mother Nature!", and a crown materializing after eating Imperial margarine. Trans fats are hydrogenated oils and they come in the form of margarine and artificial shortenings.

The current most popular margarine in America has no hydrogenated nor trans fats, yet it is very high in polyunsaturated fats. 1 tbsp (14.2 g) has 8.0 g of fat of which 2.0 g is saturated fat, 0.0 g is trans fat, 3.5 polyunsaturated fat and 3.0 g is monounsaturated fat.

Low fat diet proponents point out the need to reduce all types of fat and cite the following study, "A study on humans conducted by David Blankenhorn, M.D., and his associates (1990) compared the effects of different types of fats on the growth of atherosclerotic lesions inside the coronary arteries of people by studying the results of angiograms taken one year apart.

The study demonstrated that all three types of fat–saturated animal fat, monounsaturated (olive oil), and polyunsaturated (EFA)–were associated with a significant increase in new atherosclerotic lesions. Most importantly, the growth of these lesions did not stop when polyunsaturated fats of the w-6 type (linoleic acid) and monounsaturated fats (olive oil) were substituted for saturated fats. Only by decreasing all fat intake–including poly- and monounsaturated fats–did the lesions stop growing."

This study was refuted, however, by another study which tested the actual composition of arterial plaque of deceased humans and did not rely on angiograms. Completed in 1994 (Felton, Crook, Davies, Oliver), it studied the relation of dietary fat to the composition of human aortic plaques. The study compared the fatty-acid composition of aortic plaques with that of the serum and adipose tissue of humans that had recently died.

The fatty-acid content of the serum and adipose tissue reflects dietary intake. Positive associations were found between serum and plaque for omega 6 (r = 0.75) and omega 3 (r = 0.93, the highest association) polyunsaturated fatty acids, and monounsaturates (r = 0.70), and also between adipose tissue and plaque for omega 6 polyunsaturated fatty acids (r = 0.89), but **NO associations were found with saturated fatty acids.**

The study's findings imply a direct influence of dietary polyunsaturated fatty acids but not saturated fatty acids on aortic plaque formation and suggest that current trends favoring increased intake of polyunsaturated fatty acids should be reconsidered.

Polyunsaturated fat found in extracted seed oils (soy, safflower, cottonseed, canola, peanut, sunflower, corn, flax) are what make up arterial lesions and not saturated fat as found in grass-fed dairy products. The study also shows a positive association of monounsaturated fats and aortic plaque, albeit less than that for omega-3 or omega-6 polyunsaturated fats. This means that avocados and olive oil, which are considered natural fats must be eaten in restricted amounts or avoided altogether due to their high monounsaturated fat content and moderate polyunsaturated fat content. A medium avocado of 136 gram weight without skin or seed has 13.3 g monounsaturated fat and 2.5 g polyunsaturated fat.

The U.S. National Academy of Sciences safe range is 0.6 to 1.2 grams Omega-3 polyunsaturated fats per day for men and women. Above this safe range they warn: "While no defined intake level at which potential adverse effects of n-3 polyunsaturated fatty acids was identified, **the upper end of AMDR is based on maintaining the appropriate balance with n-6 fatty acids** and on the lack of evidence that demonstrates long-term safety, along with human in vitro studies which show **increased free-radical formation and lipid peroxidation with higher amounts of polyunsaturated fatty acids. Lipid peroxidation is thought to be a component in the development of atherosclerotic plaques.'**

The appropriate balance of n-3 to n-6 fatty acids is close to 1:1, that means n-6 or Omega-6 fatty acids also should be in the .6 to 1.2 grams maximum consumption range and not in the 5-10 gram range, which is the current AMDR.

AMDR or Acceptable Macronutrient Distribution Range is the range of intake for a particular energy source that is associated with reduced risk of chronic disease while providing intakes of essential nutrients.

Half a medium avocado has 1.25 g of polyunsaturated fat which is in the acceptable range, however this does not include the monounsaturated fats, 6.65 g, which also have been shown to be components of aortic plaque.

Even olive oil is high in unsaturated fats. One tablespoon of olive oil has 9.8 g monounsaturated fat and 1.4 g polyunsaturated fat. Compare this to one tablespoon of coconut oil which has 0.2 g polyunsaturated fat, 0.8 g monounsaturated fat and 11.7 g saturated fat.

One tablespoon of butter has 0.4 g polyunsaturated fat, 2.9 g monounsaturated fat and 7.2 g saturated fat. One tablespoon of sour cream has 0.1 g polyunsaturated fat, 0.6 g monounsaturated fat and 1.4 g saturated fat. It's healthier to use grass-fed butter, grass-fed sour cream and coconut oil which are almost entirely stable non-oxidizing saturated fats as your fat source.

THE FRAMINGHAM STUDY: "...THE MORE SATURATED FAT ONE ATE...THE LOWER THE PERSON'S SERUM CHOLESTEROL..."

The Framingham Study is one of the most famous and respected studies on heart disease and cholesterol because of its long duration. It was started in 1948 and is still in operation.

Is high cholesterol bad for you? Forty years after the start of this study of 5,000 men and women in 1948, its director, Dr. William Castelli, reluctantly admitted, "In Framingham, Massachusetts the more saturated fat one ate, the more cholesterol one ate, the more calories one ate, the lower the person's serum cholesterol. We found that the people who ate the most cholesterol, ate the most calories, weighed the least and were the most active." Those who ate the most cholesterol and saturated fat gained the least amount of weight due to being more active.

Although the study did find an association between high levels of blood cholesterol and increased likelihood of future heart attacks, the elevated cholesterol was only one of over 240 "risk factors" that were associated with increased risk of heart attacks.

If you are under 50, high cholesterol is associated with death and cardio-vascular disease i.e. heart attacks and strokes. This association was found only in young and middle aged men.

In the 30 year follow-up of the Framingham Study, high cholesterol was not predictive of heart attack at all after the age of 47. According to the Framingham Study, once a man reaches the age of 48 there is no relationship between high levels of cholesterol and dying of heart attack.

Most alarming is the fact that those whose cholesterol dropped without any intervention ran a much higher risk of heart attack than those whose cholesterol increased. The significantly increased risk of dying from heart disease and stroke in those whose cholesterol decreased is so contrary to what we have been led to believe.

HIGHER OMEGA-3 FATTY ACIDS IN GRASS-FED MILK AND CHEESE MEANS WE DON'T NEED FLAXSEED, FISH, OR COD LIVER OIL TO GET OUR OMEGA-3 FATTY ACIDS

There are 16.5 mg of omega-3 fatty acids and 16.6 mg of omega-6 fatty acids per gram of butterfat in grass-fed, pasture-raised animals (Dhiman, et al., 1999).

Three cups of grass-fed whole milk yogurt has 396 mg omega-3 and 398.4 mg omega-6. 100 grams or 3.5 ounces of grass-fed cheddar cheese has 544.5 mg omega-3 and 547.8 mg omega-6. From the 544.5 mg omega-3 fatty acids you get 87.12 mg long chain fatty acids (DHA, EPA) using the 16% conversion rate for young men. Healthy young women can convert omega-3 fatty acids at a 36% rate which would give them 196.02 mg long chain fatty acids (DHA, EPA) in 100 grams grass-fed cheddar cheese.

There is a 1:1 ratio of omega-6 to omega-3 fatty acids in grass-fed dairy products. This is the ideal ratio of essential fatty acids or EFAs according to Jo Robinson who co-authored the book *The Omega Diet* with Dr. Artemis Simopoulos in 1999. The book sites many studies showing that when your diet contains roughly equal amounts of these two fats, you will have a lower risk of cancer, cardiovascular disease, autoimmune disorders, allergies, obesity, diabetes, dementia, and various other mental disorders.

The safe range set by the Institute of Medicine (IOM) of the U.S. National Academy of Sciences for Omega-3 fatty acids is 0.6 to 1.2 grams per day for men and women. Eating the above dairy products (Three cups of grass-fed whole milk yogurt and 3.5 ounces of cheddar cheese) from a grass-fed source will give you 940.5 mg omega-3 which is within the safe range.

New research shows that cows that graze at relatively high altitudes may produce the healthiest milk of all. Compared with lowland grazers, milk from high altitude Swiss grazers (3700-6200 ft) has more

CLA (Conjugated linoleic acid). CLA has been shown, by numerous studies, to prevent cancer.

Plants growing in higher altitudes have more omega-3 fatty acids, fats which solidify at lower temperatures than other fats, and therefore act as a form of anti-freeze (Hauswirth et al, 2004). Swiss alpine cheese contained 4 times more omega-3 compared with commercially available English cheddar and showed a significantly lower amount of omega-6.

Some health advocates recommend taking flax seed oil to get your daily omega fatty acids at a dosage of two grams of organic, cold-pressed flaxseed oil and five grams of organic, cold-pressed, high linoleic sesame oil a day.

2 grams of flaxseed oil has 1,097 mg of omega-3 fatty acids. There is 2174 mg omega-6 in 5 grams sesame oil. This is an approximately 2 to 1 ratio of omega-6 to omega-3 fatty acids if we round the figures. Our results eating grass-fed dairy products was; 940.5 mg omega-3 and 946.2 mg omega-6 giving us an even better, 1 to 1 ratio.

Some authors recommend taking 10 gm of raw, organic pumpkin seeds per day but that will give you problems with the phytic acid found in the whole seed.

Most authors agree that using food sources which, combined, deliver the omega-6 to omega-3 oil in a 1:1 to 2.5:1 ratio is very important. Ratios beyond either end of this range do not appear to help tissue cell oxygenation. Omega-6 is not a 'bad' but a good fat if derived from grass-fed, whole fat dairy products. The body needs the right balance of undamaged omega-6 and undamaged omega-3 (anywhere between the ratios 1:1 and 2.5:1) to function properly. Undamaged means un-oxidized. All extracted seed oils are damaged by oxidation when exposed to the air. Grass-fed dairy fats as found in whole yogurt and cheese are saturated and thus not oxidizable.

Other authors recommend taking a daily dose of 1 or 1.5 tablespoons of flaxseed oil which would give you 7.2-10.8 grams Omega-3 fatty acids per day (1 tablespoon for women weighing 100 lbs. and 1.5 tablespoon for men weighing 150 lbs.).

Other authors even recommend taking 2 tablespoons of flaxseed oil per 100 pound body weight which would give 21.6 grams of omega-3 fatty acids per 3 tablespoons of flaxseed oil in a 150 pound person. All these recommendations to take extracted seed oils in high doses well above the Dietary Reference Intake or DRI is dangerous due to free-radical formation and lipid peroxidation of extracted polyunsaturated oils.

The DRI (Dietary Reference Intake) for men, 14 to over 70, is 1.6 grams Omega-3 per day and for women 14 to over 70 the DRI is 1.1 grams Omega-3 per day.

The DRI or Dietary Reference Intake is set by the Institute of Medicine (IOM) of the U.S. National Academy of Sciences and is used by the United States and Canada. The DRI nutrient tables give this warning about over-consuming omega-3s,

"While no defined intake level at which potential adverse effects of n-3 polyunsaturated fatty acids was identified, the upper end of AMDR (Acceptable Macronutrient Distribution Range) is based on maintaining the appropriate balance with n-6 fatty acids and on the lack of evidence that demonstrates long-term safety, along with human in vitro studies which show increased free-radical formation and lipid peroxidation with higher amounts of polyunsaturated fatty acids. Lipid peroxidation is thought to be a component of the development of **atherosclerotic plaques.**"

The DRI for omega-6 or linoleic acid is 17 grams per day for males 19-50 and 14 grams for those over 50. For women the DRI for omega-6 is 12 grams per day for those 19-50 years of age and 11 grams for those over 50. Why is this figure so high given that omega-6 fatty acids have been proven to be components of arterial plaque and are known to need a 1 to 1 ratio with Omega-3 fatty acids in order to be health giving?

During the turn of the last century, 1900, heart disease was practically unknown in the United States even tho consumption of butter and whole milk cheese was high. Only until the introduction of extracted seed oils and hydrogenated seed oil margarine and shortening did heart disease and cancer start to escalate. From about 1920 to 1960, the incidence of heart disease rose precipitously to become America's number one killer. During the same period butter consumption plummeted from eighteen pounds, per person per year, to four. By 1975, we were eating one-fourth the amount of butter eaten in 1900 and ten times the amount of margarine. Given the evidence that unsaturated fats form atherosclerotic plaques, it appears that vegetable oils and hydrogenated vegetable oils in the form of margarine and shortening is the cause of the epidemic of heart disease in the United States.

The safe range the National Academy of Sciences states is 0.6 to 1.2 grams of Omega-3 fatty acids per day for men and women.

Overdosing on omega-3 fats in the form of taking flaxseed oil, fish oil or cod liver oil may cause atherosclerotic plaques to develop. Flax-seed oil has a whopping 7,196 mg omega-3 fatty acids per tablespoon. There are 4,767 mg of omega-3 fatty acids in 1 tablespoon of salmon fish oil. Cod liver oil has 2,664 mg of omega-3 fatty acids in 1 table-spoon. Even consuming fish, especially fatty fish, has its risk; half a fillet (198 gms) of wild Coho salmon, a moderately fatty fish, has 2,918 milligrams of omega-3 fatty acids.

THE FRENCH PARADOX PHENOMENON

The French generally eat three times as much saturated animal fat as Americans do, and only about a third as many die of heart attacks according to an article in Salon magazine (Fraser, 2000). French food is high in saturated fat and cholesterol; full-fat cheese and yogurt, but-ter, bread, fresh fruits and vegetables (often grilled or sautéed), small portions of meat (more often fish or chicken than red meat), wine, and dark chocolate, yet they have a much lower incidence of heart disease than do Americans.

The French enjoy their food without guilt and they eat in a struc-tured, communal, slowed-down, leisurely, family-oriented manner. They also eat smaller portions and do not over-eat, or eat too fast like Americans.

Nor do the French eat between meals or in other words don't snack on junk foods. The French love local, high quality produce and dairy products versus the factory farm produced fare of Americans. French dairies are more likely to raise their cows on pasture, resulting in naturally high levels of conjugated omega-3 fatty acids which are known to be cancer preventing.

French people don't care about low-fat, low-carb, low-calorie, they just enjoy their rich whole milk cheeses, yogurts and creams in mod-eration and don't obsess over calories and omega-3's.

They don't sell fake "sweet and low" cream or artificial sweetener in France and they are not obsessed with high-priced nutritional supplements because they get their vitamins and minerals from real, whole food.

Their meat consumption is in small portions and they prefer bistros and sidewalk cafes rather than all you can eat smorgasbords and fast food hamburger chains.

The French as a nation indicate that saturated fat and cholesterol are not the cause of heart disease. Look at the statistics: France has 39.8 heart disease deaths per 100,000 people. The USA has 106.5 per 100,000 people, about 2 and 1/2 times more than France. SOURCE: Heart disease deaths per 100,000 population (1995-1998) World Health Organization.

Using the more recent statistics (2004) of the American Heart Association, France had 208 total heart disease deaths per 100,000 compared to 348 for the United States for men age 35 to 74. The figure is higher because this is just for older men, who are the most likely to die from heart disease.

Now what about China? Is not the China study supposed to prove that a vegan diet is healthy?

According to the American Heart Association's 2004 data, using WHO statistics, China has more heart disease than the United States and it is even higher in rural China than urban China: 413 deaths per 100,000 rural and 398 heart disease deaths urban, compared to 348 per 100,000 in the USA.

The Chinese and especially the rural Chinese (too poor to eat meat) are supposed to have a heart healthy diet yet they have more heart disease than the United States.

The French eat lots of saturated fat and cholesterol but they have the lowest rate of cardiovascular disease deaths among industrialized nations.

The China Study is being referred to as conclusive evidence that any amount of dietary animal protein increases one's risk of cancer and other degenerative health conditions. This study did not take into account critical factors that determine the suitability of animal products for human consumption and health.

How does human health respond to eating grass fed, naturally raised dairy products vs. factory farmed dairy products? Without searching for and considering the answers to these questions, how can we make such a bold conclusion that eating any amount of animal protein causes disease?

Eating factory farmed animal products is harmful to human health. However, eating moderate amounts of grass-fed animal foods like organic, raw yogurt, kefir, cottage cheese, cheese, sour cream and butter is essential to health.

The latest April, 2011 WHO figures show that France has lower heart disease deaths than Japan, the US and China: France .30% (of the total population die of heart disease), Japan .34%, US .55% and China .58%. The figure was calculated dividing the number of deaths from heart disease by the total population of the country.

The French have the healthier diet and lifestyle because they have lower heart disease, which is the #1 killer worldwide.

France has a 29.2 death rate for coronary heart disease per 100,000 population making it second only to the Pacific island of Kiribati according to worldlifeexpectancy.com which uses, "the most recent data from these primary sources: WHO, World Bank, UNESCO, CIA and individual country databases for global health and causes of death. We use the CDC, NIH and individual state and county databases for verification and supplementation for USA data." They combine all the statistics from the major sources which gives you an average of all data.

Kiribati is a poor country and unfortunately has the 40th highest stroke rate out of 192 countries with 141.5 deaths per 100,000 making it unwise to follow their diet and lifestyle. The top cause of death in France is lung cancer due to smoking.

According to the WHO, "CVDs (Cardio-Vascular-Diseases) are the number one cause of death globally: more people die annually from CVDs than from any other cause.

An estimated 17.1 million people died from CVDs in 2004, representing 29% of all global deaths. Of these deaths, an estimated 7.2

million were due to coronary heart disease and 5.7 million were due to stroke.

Low- and middle-income countries are disproportionally affected: 82% of CVD deaths take place in low- and middle-income countries and occur almost equally in men and women. By 2030, almost 23.6 million people will die from CVDs, mainly from heart disease and stroke. These are projected to remain the single leading causes of death."

WHERE TO FIND GRASS-FED, PASTURE-RAISED ORGANIC DAIRY PRODUCTS

The new USDA ORGANIC RULES for dairy products 2010 are: "Animals must graze pasture during the grazing season, which must be at least 120 days per year; Animals must obtain a minimum of 30 percent dry matter intake from grazing pasture during the grazing season; Producers must have a pasture management plan and manage pasture as a crop to meet the feed requirements for the grazing animals and to protect soil and water quality; and, Livestock are exempt from the 30 percent dry matter intake requirements during the finish feeding period, not to exceed 120 days. Livestock must have access to pasture during the finishing phase."

Clover Stornetta is organic and pasture raised and available in California, Arizona and Nevada. Both their natural and organic milk is pasture raised. Clover Stornetta products are available at all Whole Foods Markets and many local, small groceries.

Straus family creamery in Marshall California is pasture raised and is available in Northern and Southern California. Phoenix, Arizona and even Portland, Oregon but not Las Vegas, Nevada Whole Foods Markets, Safeways and smaller grocers carry it.

Organic Valley dairy products are pasture-raised and available all over the United States. In upstate New York buy Ronnybrook Farms milk and products, a small dairy (not organic, but pesticide, hormone and antibiotic-free) that also packages in glass and uses humane, sustainable practices.

The organic milk Wal-Mart sells under its own label; Great Value comes from Aurora Organic Dairy, which also supplies Safeway,

Costco, Target and Wild Oats with their store brands of organic milk.

John Mackay, chief executive of Whole Foods Market, the largest organic food supermarket chain in the US, toured Aurora's Platteville farm and found it to be "unacceptable" and "not up to our standards."

Aurora Organic Dairy is a huge corporation and is really just factory confined area dairy farming using organic soy and corn grains instead of gmo pesticide raised grains. Healthy, natural milk is from pasture-raised cows not confined grain fed cows.

It's important to note that Aurora supplies milk for many other private labels including Costco's "Kirkland Signature," Safeway's "O" organics brand, Publix's "High Meadows", Giant's "Natures Promise," and Wild Oats organic milk. To find real organic pasteurized milk you have to avoid the giant corporate chain stores and go to Whole Foods Market or a small, local grocer.

Organic Pasture's raw milk dairy out of Fresno does not sell its dairy products at Whole Foods Market but it can be found at smaller local natural food stores, local grocers and farmer's markets. Claravale raw milk is sold in glass bottles at many independent natural food stores and grocers throughout California but not at Whole Foods.

If you have very young children or you are elderly it is best to use fermented, raw, grass-fed organic dairy products like yogurt, kefir and cheese. The lactic acid kills any harmful bacteria.

Organic Pastures raw dairy farm on its website states that, "The consequences of drinking contaminated raw milk can be very serious, especially for some young children and those that have damaged, immature immune systems or certain medical conditions. Like all unprocessed and raw food, raw milk is never guaranteed to be perfectly safe and free of harmful bacteria."

As a graduate student in Wisconsin, Mokua hypothesized that high levels of lactic acid in amasi, a traditional fermented milk were protecting children from illness caused by pathogenic bacteria. Raw milk actually has little lactic acid, but when it's cultured with a high lactic acid bacteria culture, the culture can protect against the growth of pathogens.

Mokua took on E. coli because of E. coli 0157:H7, the infamous bacteria that loves to lurk in hamburgers, spinach, and cookie dough.

Mokua examined the ability of amasi to kill E. coli bacteria in partial fulfillment of his Master's degree. For his study, Mokua acquired an amasi culture from his hometown in Kenya. He purchased some milk and commercial yogurt and fermented some of the Wisconsin milk as amasi and set some aside as a "control" milk in the experiment. He then inoculated the yogurt, amasi, and regular milk (plus another control item) with the E. coli bacteria.

We would not expect regular milk to kill E. coli. Raw milk does not even kill it consistently and thoroughly. However, amasi did kill the pathogen and it killed it faster than did the cultured yogurt product.

Amasi killed (reduced from 3000 colony counts to 100) the pathogenic E. coli. in 2 hours, the commercial yogurt killed the E. coli in 4 hours.

The results are fairly compelling and do fit into a larger research school of the effect of cultured dairy on the survivability of pathogens.

In this case, the primary difference between regular commercial yogurt and the amasi was the amount of lactic acid bacteria.

Lactic acid bacteria, including lactobacillus, is recognized as an important probiotic in human health and amasi happens to be loaded with it.

The lactic acid bacteria in amasi helped protect the amasi itself from an assault by pathogens. It can do the same in your gut should you draw a bad card at your dinner table and consume pathogenic bacteria. Of course, as in all of life's risks, there are no guarantees.

Raw milk can be used to make yogurt and other fermented dairy products because the bad bacteria are eliminated by the lactic acid in the yogurt.

Drinking raw milk without fermenting it is unhealthy because the lacto-bacteria pre-digest the lactose and protein allowing easy digestion.

I have experimented drinking raw milk and the result was an ear ache, a runny nose and neck lymph node pain and congestion. Raw milk yogurt produces none of these effects.

Children adapt to drinking milk as young children but this is in part the cause of all the childhood diseases. Milk needs to be cultured to render it digestible.

PASTEURIZATION VERSUS RAW MILK

There is evidence of cattle domestication in Mesopotamia as early as 8000 B.C.E. or about 10,000 years ago. Milking of dairy cows did not become a major part of Sumerian civilization until approximately 3000 B.C.E. or about 5,000 years ago. The milk they used was raw.

In 1624 the first cows were brought to the Plymouth colony in America. The Jesuit Priest, Eusebio Kino, introduced cattle to Baja California in 1679 as part of the missionary effort to establish mission settlements. Milk became a blessing to missionaries in time of need. During a food shortage in 1772, Junipero Serra stated that "...milk from the cows and some vegetables from the garden have been [our] chief subsistence." In 1776, at Mission San Gabriel (south of Pasadena California) Father Font wrote that "The cows are very fat and they give much and rich milk, which they (Native American women at the mission) make cheese and very good butter." Again using raw milk.

Until the middle of the 1800s most Americans and Europeans, drank most of their (raw) milk fermented, soured into the yogurt-like food known as clabbered milk. Clabbered milk is raw milk that has been left out at room temperature to ferment naturally by the bacteria in the air. Clabbered milk and other fermented dairy beverages were all called "milk." This is also true of traditional dairy-based cultures throughout the world that have survived into the twentieth century.

Fermented milk products, fresh cheese and butter were the core of the traditional colonial American diet and drinking fresh, sweet milk was confined to farmers, children and milkmaids. Drinking fresh milk did not begin to become popular in America until around 1850, when the need arose for a breast milk substitute and a food for weaned infants. Many of those demanding fresh milk were immigrants from Europe, where a similar transition was occurring.

Women moving to the big cities found poverty, poor sanitation, inadequate nutrition and long hours in factories. These unhealthy conditions of big city life rendered more and more new mothers unable to breast-feed, and thus the need for a mother's milk substitute. In addition poorly nourished, just weaned toddlers needed a nutritious food.

Distillery dairies, or dairies that fed their cows the waste products of the alcoholic beverage industry, grew in tandem with the growth of the cities. Distillery dairies, which were unsanitary and fed the cow's un-nutritious waste products from the distilling of grains, supplied up to three-quarters of city milk.

Alcohol production results in large amounts of processed grain. Disposing of distillery waste in big cities was a major expense so feeding the swill to dairy cows penned nearby made economic sense. To get grass-eating ruminants to eat the smelly feed, farmers would first cut off all food and water, then give them salt to induce thirst. Eventually they were given cold slop until they grew accustomed to it, after which they could be fed with hot swill right from the alcohol stills.

Cows confined to crowded, reeking, manure-filled pens, suffered numerous diseases and debilitating injuries. The milk of these abused cows was deficient in calcium and lacked its normal self-protective bacteria.

It was called blue milk due to its lack of butterfat which is yellow white in color. Butter or cheese could not be made from this artificial, factory made milk. Greed and ignorance turned the natural health giving food called raw milk from grass-fed cows into a disease causing nutrition deficient product.

By 1880 not only children in the cities but the adults too began to consume fresh milk. Around 1910, many American cities had imposed a pasteurization requirement due to the unsanitary conditions of the distillery dairies due largely to the work of Nathan Straus, who made a fortune as co-owner of New York's Macy's department stores and spent decades promoting pasteurization across America and Europe. Using his considerable wealth, Straus set up and subsidized the first of many "milk depots" in New York City to provide low-cost pasteurized milk.

In 1889, Newark, New Jersey doctor Henry Coit, MD urged the creation of a Medical Milk Commission to oversee or "certify" production of milk for cleanliness, finally getting one formed in 1893. After years of effort, raw, unpasteurized milk was again safe and available for public consumption, but it cost up to four times the price of uncertified milk.

Pasteurized and certified "raw" milks peacefully co-existed for about 50 years until in 1944 when a media smear campaign was launched (by the giant factory farm dairies of course) to spark fear at the very thought of consuming raw milk.

Pasteurization is simply a quick fix that allows corporate factory farms to profit from the sales of cheaply produced milk. Instead of using costly, safe, sterile handling procedures of raw milk and allowing the cows to graze pasture versus being confined to excrement laden yards, the factory farms devised a quick fix, to create the illusion of germ free milk in order to maximize profits. By 1940 fluid milk was a staple in the American diet and by 1950, most milk was pasteurized.

The first pasteurization test was completed by Louis Pasteur and Claude Bernard in April 1862 and it was done on alcoholic beverages not milk. The process was originally conceived as a way of preventing wine and beer from souring, but in 1886 Franz von Soxhlet from Germany suggested that pasteurization be used for milk and other beverages.

Pasteur described germs as non-changeable. We know today, from the use of Darkfield Microscopes that microorganisms are pleomorphic and that they can change; a virus can become a bacterium which can mutate into a yeast or fungus. Bechamp discovered the pleomorphic nature of germs, and then Bernard described the "milieu" or environment that caused those changes in the germ.

Bernard is the one responsible for our theories today on pH and how the nature of the microorganisms change as the body moves from an alkaline pH to an acidic pH. On his deathbed, Pasteur changed his mind, saying that Bernard was right; "the Terrain is everything, the Germ is nothing." The germ theory of disease has it backwards because if the body is clean and the immune system is functioning well, disease cannot occur even if the person is in contact with contagious, sick people.

Dr Lanctôt points out that typhoid, coli bacillus and tuberculosis are not killed by pasteurization and there have been a good number of salmonella epidemics traced to pasteurized milk. Dr Lanctôt also points out that pasteurization destroys milk's intrinsic germicidal properties and healthy enzymes like lactase and that 50% of milk's calcium is unassimilable by the body after pasteurization.

Concerning the calcium availability in pasteurized milk compared to raw milk, less favorable calcium balances where found in adults using pasteurized milk than with fresh milk (raw milk). In addition milk from cows kept in the barn for five months gave less favorable calcium balances than did "fresh milk (raw milk)", the herd milk from the college dairy (Kramer, Latzke and Shaw, 1928).

Studies have shown that harmful bacteria are not the only thing destroyed by the heat of pasteurization: delicate proteins, enzymes, immune factors, hormones, vitamins, mineral availability, all undergo definite changes during the heating process. Not even the public health agencies dispute this fact.

When man-made nutrients like vitamin D must be added back in to replace those destroyed by heat, it's a no brainer; the quality of the milk has suffered. There are hundreds of factors and components present in raw milk, known and unknown, that synergistically create a whole, natural food.

Pasteurization is supposed to kill the pathogenic bacteria in milk. Sally Fallon from the Weston Price Foundation compiled a list of U.S. government documented outbreaks of food-borne illness from pasteurized milk for Ted Elkins, Deputy Director for Maryland's Office of Food Protection and Consumer Health Services.

Pasteurized milk caused outbreaks of illness:
1945 — 1,492 cases for the year in the US
1945 — 1 outbreak, 300 cases in Phoenix, Arizona.
1945 — Several outbreaks, 468 cases of gastroenteritis, 9 deaths, in Great Bend, Kansas
1976 — Outbreak of Yersinia enterocolitica in 36 children, 16 of whom had appendectomies, due to pasteurized chocolate milk
1978 — 1 outbreak, 68 cases in Arizona
1982 — over 17,000 cases of Yersinia enterocolitica in Memphis, TN
1982 — 172 cases, with over 100 hospitalized from a three-Southern-state area.
1983 — 1 outbreak, 49 cases of Listeriosis in Massachusetts
1984 — August, 1 outbreak S. typhimurium, approximately 200 cases,

at one plant in Melrose Park, IL

1984—November, 1 outbreak S. typhimurium, at same plant in Melrose Park, IL

1985—March, 1 outbreak, 16,284 confirmed cases, at same plant in Melrose Park, IL

1985—197,000 cases of antimicrobial-resistant Salmonella infections from one dairy in California

1985—1,500+ cases, Salmonella culture confirmed, in Northern Illinois

1987—Massive outbreak of over 16,000 culture-confirmed cases of antimicrobial-resistant Salmonella typhimurium traced to pasteurized milk in Georgia

1993—2 outbreaks statewide, 28 cases Salmonella infection

1994—3 outbreaks, 105 cases, E. Coli & Listeria in California

1993-1994—outbreak of Salmonella enteritidis in over 200 due to pasteurized ice cream in Minnesota, South Dakota and Wisconsin

1995—1 outbreak, 3 cases in California

1995—outbreak of Yersinia enterocolitica in 10 children, 3 hospitalized due to post-pasteurization contamination

1996—2 outbreaks Campylobactor and Salmonella, 48 cases in California

1997—2 outbreaks, 28 cases Salmonella in California

"What consumers need to realize, first of all," said Sally Fallon Morell, president of the Weston A. Price Foundation, "is that the incidence of foodborne illnesses from dairy products, whether pasteurized or not, is extremely low. For the 14-year period that the authors examined, there was an average of 315 illnesses a year from all dairy products for which the pasteurization status was known. Of those, there was an average of 112 illnesses each year attributed to all raw dairy products and 203 associated with pasteurized dairy products."

"In comparison, there are almost 24,000 foodborne illnesses reported each year on average. Whether pasteurized or not, dairy products are simply not a high risk product."

In a response to a Freedom of Information request, the Centers for Disease Control provided data on raw milk outbreaks 1993-2005. In this report, CDC listed NO, repeat ZERO, cases of foodborne illness from raw milk caused by listeria during the period, yet pasteurized milk looking at the chart above did cause listeria.

Factory-farm dairy animals kept knee deep in excrement and fed a diet of GMO corn and soy have 300 times more pathogenic bacteria in their digestive tracts than cattle that are allowed to openly graze in pastures.

Pasteurization was never intended for milk, it was invented for beer and wine. Pasteurization was adopted to cover up the horrible conditions of confined pen, grain-fed milk factories. How different this is from the ideal of contented cows grazing in lush green fields. Dr. Weston Price traveled the globe looking for isolated groups of people who had maintained their traditional way of food production and did not rely on civilized, processed foods. In an isolated mountain valley in Switzerland Dr. Price found a group of people with virtually no tooth decay.

In the Loetschental Valley in Switzerland only 0.3% of all teeth were affected with tooth decay. The diet of the people of the Loetschental Valley consists of carefully processed sourdough rye bread, summer raw milk cheese (about as large as the slice of bread), which is eaten with fresh milk of goats or cows. Meat is only eaten once a week.

The samples of food analyzed for nutritional content were found to be much higher than the average samples of commercial dairy products in America and Europe, and even in the lower, non mountainous areas of Switzerland.

It is clear why they have healthy bodies and sound teeth. The average total fat-soluble activator (fat soluble vitamins A, D, E and K-2) and mineral intake of calcium and phosphorus of these children far exceed that of the daily intake of the average American child. There was no need for doctors, dentists or policeman in this traditional dairy based community.

Is milk mucus forming or is it the pasteurization or cooking of milk that makes it mucus forming? Raw milk and raw dairy by-products contain the enzyme lactase which helps us digest lactose. People who are lactose intolerant are lacking lactase so they can't digest the lactose. This is why so many people who are lactose-intolerant have no problems drinking raw milk. Excessive mucus production is a common sign of an allergic reaction.

Nutritionist, David Getoff of the Price-Pottenger Foundation says, "Well, we shouldn't say raw milk, we should say milk if it's raw and cooked milk instead of pasteurized (because you are basically bringing it up to the temperature that is starting to cook it). When you do that you destroy all the enzymes that are in the milk, and you also denature some of the proteins.

Pasteurization alters the milk. A lot of people are intolerant of some of the changes that have occurred in this food that otherwise wouldn't have bothered them.

From my own impromptu research with a couple of thousand students and patients over many years, approximately 8 out of every 10 people who have a problem with milk or dairy, do not have the problem when it is consumed RAW.

Pasteurized dairy causes one of a variety of problems depending on the person, and people do not realize that they do not have a problem with raw milk, they only have a problem after it's been pasteurized and homogenized. So milk is not necessarily the issue. A lot of people know that they are lactose intolerant which is the sugar that occurs in milk.

Lactose intolerance is not a milk allergy. It doesn't mean milk is not good for them. It simply means that the milk sugar, which is called lactose, can't be properly assimilated by the body because the lactase enzyme is either not there or is in an insufficient amount and therefore causes a problem. Lo and behold Mother Nature knows that the human body generally doesn't do well with lactose. So she put plenty of lactase into the milk so it wouldn't cause a problem, but we kill it all by pasteurizing the milk. Most people who are lactose intolerant can handle raw milk (as long as they don't use it to cook with)."

Raw milk products like homemade yogurt, cottage cheese and cheese are healthier than pasteurized milk yogurt, cottage cheese and cheese because they don't lose any nutrients or enzymes. Pasteurized, uncultured fluid milk can be problematic causing excess mucus formation and the resultant cold symptoms. Pasteurized cheeses, yogurt and sour cream are cultured by bacteria so they are less likely to cause problems with mucus formation.

The French love raw milk cheeses. Raw milk and especially raw milk cheeses are considered the standard for high quality dairy products in France. Many French cuisine traditionalists consider pasteurized cheeses almost a sacrilege. Traditional French cheeses have been made from raw milk for hundreds of years. The bacteria found in raw milk are essential to the flavors of many cheeses.

"Cheese is a natural, living animal," says Joe Manacusso, the cheese buyer for Citarella in New York City. "It shouldn't be treated with heat and plastic the way it is in this country. That compromises the product. Yes, there is a small factor of contamination from raw-milk cheeses, but the French have been eating this way for hundreds of years without much consequence."

Raw milk dispensing machines are found in front of supermarkets in the middle of France and in Italy too you can find raw milk vending machines. The most famous (and delicious) French cheeses are made with raw milk. Camembert, Brie, Roquefort, and all of the best of these cheeses are made with raw milk. Raw milk cheeses are sold in grocery stores and little corner markets all across France.

The best brands of butter that are served in the top-starred restaurants are made from raw milk. Crème fraîche is a cultured cream which is made somewhat like yogurt producing a tangy and unbelievably rich product. In France you find regular pasteurized cream, but the best cream is made from raw milk and has a richer flavor and texture.

Of the 100-150 raw milk cheeses available in France, three disappear each year, meaning around 40 have become extinct in the last decade. France is long known as a country of avid cheese-eaters, with more than 1,000 varieties and overall cheese consumption is on the rise in France, but industrially-made products are out selling traditional farm-crafted varieties. When a farm-crafted cheese business shuts down cows are sold and pastures planted with corn, which pollutes the lands, so keeping traditional cheeses alive helps to create sustainable development.

MARGARINE: THE FIRST MAN-MADE FAT

Margarine is anything but the healthy, heart-friendly alternative to butter, it is a highly processed, chemical laden, artificial concoction.

In 1989, benzene, a petroleum-based solvent and known carcinogen, was found in Perrier mineral water in a mean concentration of fourteen parts per billion. Perrier was removed from supermarket shelves.

The first process in the manufacture of margarine is the

extraction of the oils from the seeds, and this is usually done using a similar to benzene petroleum-based solvent called hexane. Although the solvent is then boiled off, this stage of the process still leaves about ten parts per million of the solvents in the product. That is 700 times as much as fourteen parts per billion. The EPA regulates n-hexane under the Clean Air Act (CAA) and designated n-hexane as a hazardous air pollutant in 1994.

In 2010 it was reported that an employee of Wintek Corporation in China, a company that manufactures touch screen components, died in August 2009 due to hexane poisoning. Hexane was used as a replacement for alcohol for cleaning the screens. Reports suggest up to 137 Chinese employees required treatment for hexane poisoning.

An ABC Foreign Correspondent episode covertly interviewed several women who had been in the hospital for over six months. The women claimed that they were exposed to hexane while manufacturing iPhone hardware.

These refined oils like soy, cottonseed and corn then go through more than ten other processes: degumming, bleaching, hydrogenation, neutralization, fractionation, deodorization, emulsification, interesterification that includes high heat treatment with a solution of caustic soda; the use of nickel, a metal that is known to cause cancer, as a catalyst, with up to fifty parts per million of the nickel left in the product and the addition of antioxidants such as butylated hydroxyanisol (E320). These antioxidants are usually petroleum based and are widely believed to cause cancer.

The hydrogenation process, that solidifies the oils so that they are spreadable, produces trans fatty acids that rarely occur in nature. Even pressed olive oil if used at frying temperatures can cause problems.

Margarine is a toxic nightmare but also remember that other shortenings made the same way are put in many different processed foods and you don't even know you are eating trans fats until you read the label closely and it says partially hydrogenated fats or vegetable shortening (Crisco etc.) on the label.

Hydrogenated trans fats became the healthy alternative to butter fat which was demonized as high in cholesterol.

In 1987 the NHI or National Institute of Health, a governmental institution, declared that 25% of the American population had high cholesterol. All those with high cholesterol would be placed on a strict diet for 3 months and if that didn't work then drugs would be prescribed.

Coincidentally, the first statin cholesterol reducing drugs were released that same year. This was the biggest medical intervention in the history of the United States, yet it was never debated sufficiently and was quietly issued without much fanfare.

This further solidified the myth that cholesterol had to be reduced to save people from the epidemic of heart disease.

MAKING RAW MILK YOGURT, CLABBERED MILK, YOGURT CHEESE, CREAM CHEESE, RICOTTA AND MOZZARELLA CHEESE

RAW YOGURT: 1. You will need one half cup of plain, unsweetened, non-fruited yogurt at the supermarket and one gallon of raw milk. Or one quarter cup of yogurt and 1 quart of raw milk. **2.** Mix the yogurt with the milk, mashing the yogurt solids into a liquid and stir it in a circle 8 motion until well mixed. **3.** Heat the milk to 110 Fahrenheit or 43 Centigrade using a kitchen thermometer to be sure. **4.** Place the liquid in a container, preferable glass and cover it with some blankets or place in an ice chest to keep it warm so the bacteria can do their work at the correct temperature. **5.** It will turn to yogurt overnight, so give it enough time to curd. If you make it at night it will be ready by morning. If you make it in the morning just wait until the next day to be sure. Place it in the refrigerator to keep it fresh. Save the top creamy layer in a cup, so it can be eaten a little at a time or make cream cheese (see below). Using your homemade raw yogurt to act as the starter for the next batch won't work because it's not as strong a culture as the original. Try different brands of unsweetened plain yogurt as the starter culture because each one uses slightly different bacteria. A more liquid type yogurt is usually less acidic than a thick, solid type yogurt.

CLABBERED MILK: Take raw milk and let it sit at room temperature for two days or so. In warmer weather the milk will curdle faster. Keep the lid off so the bacteria in the air can enter the milk. Once a curd forms you can scrape off the sour cream on top and place it in a separate plate to be eaten a little at a time, since it's so rich. For the next batch save a cup to inoculate the next batch of milk so it will curd faster.

YOGURT CHEESE: Put your homemade yogurt in a sieve and let it drain out the whey overnight. Save the whey liquid to make mozzarella cheese.

CREAM CHEESE: The top part of the yogurt will be all cream. Skim this off, place in a sieve and let it drain overnight to make cream cheese.

MOZZARELLA: Take two cups of the acidic whey you saved from making yogurt cheese and add it to one quart (one liter) of raw milk. Slowly heat it in a pan until it is hot, but not too hot to touch which is around 110 degrees Fahrenheit or 43 Centigrade. Metal kitchen thermometers can be found for around 5 dollars to be sure about the temperature. A temperature over 118 Fahrenheit or 48 Centigrade will kill the natural enzymes in raw milk. Stir slowly until the curds form, which can be grabbed in your hand and formed into a ball. Squeeze the whey out by pressing it with your hand in a sieve.

RICOTTA: Same as mozzarella but add 1 quart or 1 liter whey per quart or liter raw milk.

VEGAN AND SEMI-VEGETARIAN DIETS

THE PROBLEM WITH A VEGAN DIET

A nationwide poll conducted in April 2006 by Harris Interactive reported that 1.4% of the American population is vegan (eat no meat, fish, dairy, or eggs). Another survey was conducted by Harris Interactive by telephone within the United States on behalf of the Vegetarian Resource Group, April, 2011 and found that approximately 5% of the country, nearly 15 million say that they never eat meat, fish, seafood, or poultry. About half of these vegetarians are also vegan so you get the figure of about 2.5%, up 1.1 % since 2006. Vegan diets are growing in popularity today among teenagers and youth, especially females.

The most well known problem of the vegan diet is lack of vitamin B-12. Vegans typically have lower plasma vitamin B-12 concentrations, higher prevalence of vitamin B-12 deficiency, and higher concentrations of plasma homocysteine. Elevated homocysteine has been considered a risk factor for cardiovascular disease or CVD and osteoporotic bone fractures.

Vitamin B-12 deficiency can produce abnormal neurologic and psychiatric symptoms that include ataxia, psychoses, paresthesia, disorientation, dementia, mood and motor disturbances, and difficulty with concentration.

In addition, children may experience apathy and failure to thrive, and macrocytic anemia is a common feature at all ages. Macrocytic is from the Greek words meaning "large cell". A macrocytic class of anemia is an anemia or blood, with an insufficient concentration of hemoglobin, in which the erythrocytes are larger than their normal volume.

In addition to vitamin B-12 vegan diets tend to be lower in calories, protein, saturated fat, cholesterol, long-chain n–3 (omega-3) fatty acids, vitamin D, calcium, zinc, and vitamin B-12.

Dr. Weston Price found no cultures, that were isolated from modern civilization, that did not eat some type of animal food, and he supposed that none existed. It is only in the mind of some radical vegetarians that veganism is created theoretically without any relation to the real world.

In Nutrition and Physical Degeneration by Dr. Weston Price (can be downloaded free on the internet), Chapter 16 states that vitamin D is not found in plants and must be sought in an animal food, "There is a misapprehension with regard to the possibility that humans may obtain enough of the vitamin D group of activators from our modern plant foods or from sunshine. This is due to the belief viosterol or similar products by other names, derived by exposing ergosterol to ultraviolet light, offer all of the nutritional factors involved in the vitamin D group. I have emphasized that there are known to be at least eight D factors that have been definitely isolated and twelve that have been reported as partially isolated.

Coffin has recently reported relative to the lack of vitamin D in common foods as follows: 1. A representative list of common foods was carefully tested, by approved technique, for their vitamin D content. 2. With the remote possibility of egg yolks, butter, cream, liver and fish it is manifestly impossible to obtain any amount of vitamin D worthy of mention from common foods. 3. Vegetables and fruits do not contain vitamin D.

It will be noted that vitamin D, which the human does not readily synthesize in adequate amounts, must be provided by foods of animal tissues or animal products. As yet I have not found a single group of primitive racial stock which was building and maintaining excellent bodies by living entirely on plant foods."

Grass-fed dairy products contain high levels of vitamin K. Weston Price used butter oil and cod liver oil to reverse dental caries. This protocol caused the dentin to remineralize and seal dental decay with a glassy finish.

In the numerous butter samples tested, "Activator X" was present only when the animals were eating rapidly growing, green grass occurring in high rainfall periods. Price found the highest concentrations of Activator-X in "the milk of several species, varying with the nutrition of the animal."

Price used the animal source foods; butter oil and cod liver oil to heal teeth so the elusive Activator-X factor was the animal derived MK-4 not the bacteria/plant derived MK-7. The MK-7 form of K2 can be produced by bacterial fermentation, natto is the highest source with sauerkraut being a minor source. MK-4 is the type that mammals synthesize for themselves.

Instead of cod liver oil, which can cause cancer, it is better to use dark yellow butter, butter oil, grass fed cheese and yogurt.

THE NUMBER OF VEGETARIANS AND VEGANS IN THE UNITED STATES OF AMERICA

A 2008 study titled "Vegetarianism in America" published by Vegetarian Times (vegetariantimes.com), shows that 3.2 percent of U.S. adults, or 7.3 million people, follow a vegetarian-based diet (a newer 2011 Harris poll found 5%). Approximately 0.5 percent, or 1 million, of those are vegans, who consume no animal products at all.

In addition, 10 percent of U.S. adults, or 22.8 million people, say they largely follow a vegetarian-inclined diet. If you add the 7.3 million strict vegetarians to the 22.8 million "flexitarians", those who eat meat a few times per week or only on weekends and holidays, you come up with the figure of 30.1 million adult Americans being vegetarian or largely vegetarian. This does not include all the children under 18 who are vegan or vegetarian.

These flexitarians are making the transition slowly to being full-time vegetarians. If a person eats some meat unknowingly or eats a little meat at a holiday feast they are still 99% vegetarian and should be considered strict vegetarians. Those who reduce their meat consumption for their health, for animal rights or the environment ought to be considered novice vegetarians also using the new flexible definition.

It's best to urge people to give up meat one day a week in the beginning and not go cold turkey. Once they taste how delicious meatless recipes can be they will find out for themselves they can live with less meat in their diet.

The poll, collected by the Harris Interactive Service Bureau and analyzed by RRC Associates, surveyed 5,050 respondents, a statistically representative sample of the total U.S. population. The survey was commissioned by Vegetarian Times. The 2008 study also indicates that of the non-vegetarians surveyed 5.2 percent, or 11.9 million people, are "definitely interested" in following a vegetarian-based diet in the future.

Of the vegetarians surveyed:
a.   59 percent are female; 41 percent are male.

b.   42.0 percent are age 18 to 34 years old; 40.7 percent are 35 to 54; and 17.4 percent are over 55.

c.   57.1 percent have followed a vegetarian diet for more than 10 years; 18 percent for 5 to 10 years; 10.8 percent for 2 to 5 years, 14.1 percent for less than 2 years.

The study also indicated that over half (54 percent) of the current vegetarians cited animal welfare as their reason for being vegetarian which is just over (53 percent) for those who say they eat a vegetarian diet to improve their overall health.

Environmental concerns were cited by 47 percent; 39 percent cited "natural approaches to wellness"; 31 percent cited food-safety concerns; 25 percent cited weight loss; and 24 percent weight mainte-nance.

Money talks, so if we follow the money we see vegetarians and vegans will be affecting the economy greatly in the coming years.

Vegetarian Times' editor in chief, Elizabeth Turner says, "The veg-etarian sector is one of the fastest-growing categories in food publish-ing. It's a dedicated group of consumers that is growing daily." Bill Harper, vice president and publisher of Vegetarian Times says, "A vast number of people are seeking to reduce their meat intake, creat-ing a rapidly growing market for all things vegetarian." Vegetarian Times, for over 30 years, has been at the forefront of the healthful-living movement, providing recipes, expert wellness information, and environmentally sound lifestyle solutions to vegetarians, vegans, and non-vegetarians.

Even in Las Vegas things are changing to a vegan point of view. All of the many restaurants in Steve Wynn's Las Vegas hotel serve vegan dishes as an alternative to the normal fare. The billionaire and former steak fanatic gave it all up after suffering from health prob-lems.

The animal rights movement got a big boost when McDonald's corporation decided they wanted to buy from those ranches that treated the animals humanely. Public pressure made the hamburger behemoth realize that it's good for their public image if they support humane treatment of farm animals. It's just a matter of time until the golden arches offers more and more vegetarian alternatives like veg-etable entrees, meatless salads and tempeh hamburgers.

THE FLEXITARIAN DIET

Flexitarian was voted most useful word of 2003 by the American Dialect Society. Flexitarians are those people who eat meat on a part-time basis.

Sir Paul McCartney is promoting the Meatless Monday campaign to raise awareness of the meat-less diet and its health promoting, animal rights respecting and ecology supporting qualities.

A flexitarian could be someone who doesn't eat meat on Monday or someone who eats meat only on holidays or at social gatherings, or maybe they order vegetarian dishes at restaurants wanting to take advantage of the health benefits of a vegetarian diet.

Some have given up red meat to reduce their chances of getting heart disease and cancer but still eat chicken and fish. There are as many types of flexitarians as there are different types of people.

The good thing is that people are making the effort to reduce their meat consumption because they know that it will help them become healthier and also will help the environment and the animals. More health benefits will be enjoyed by those who eat the least meat.

Vegetarian Times magazine now focuses less on animal activism and veganism and more on recipes with broader appeal. Carla Davis, managing editor, said the changes were made after a survey showed 70 percent of the magazine's 300,000-plus readers were flexitarians and not vegetarian or vegan.

Charles Stahler, co-director of the Baltimore-based Vegetarian Resource Group, estimates roughly 30 percent to 40 percent of the United States population (315,329,678 U.S. Bureau of the Census, February 14, 2013) occasionally seeks out vegetarian meals. That's about 95 to 126 million people just in the United States alone.

Bruce Friedrich, spokesman for PETA (People for the Ethical Treatment of Animals), doesn't see any harm in vegetarianism focusing more on food than the issues that spurred the movement, "From our perspective, if people influenced by health consequently cut back on fish and meat consumption, that helps animals. If two people cut their meat in half it helps as much as one person going completely vegetarian."

95 to 126 million people in the United States occasionally are flexitarians. If each one of them ate 50% of the meat they ate before, that would be equal to 47.5 to 63 million new full-time vegetarians or about 15-20% of the U.S. population.

If the U.S. population could all be part-time vegetarians eating half the meat they ate before, then there would be about 157 million full-time vegetarians.

The reality is that even vegetarians can't stick to strictly fruit and veggies 100% of the time. Studies have shown that nearly two out of three vegetarians don't, or can't, do it full-time.

Registered dietitian Dawn Jackson Blatner, author of *The Flexitarian Diet: The Mostly Vegetarian Way to Lose Weight, Be Healthier, Prevent Disease, and Add Years to Your Life*, published in 2008, says you can have the benefits of a vegetarian diet without having to follow all of the strict rules. Being a flexitarian is a more flexible way to be a vegetarian.

The benefits of becoming a flexitarian or a part-time vegetarian are that you'll reduce the likelihood of getting heart disease and cancer.

Your blood pressure, glucose, triglyceride, and cholesterol levels will plunge which is very good because if your cholesterol drops below 150 you will never have a heart attack.

Blatner shows that vegetarians on average weigh 15% less than non-vegetarians. Blatner estimates the average person could shed up to 30 pounds by sticking to the flexitarian diet for 6-12 months. That's great news since most people gain weight as they get older and it's nice to know that reducing your meat consumption and increasing plant foods will lower your weight.

Dr. Oz, the famous doctor with his own show, thanks to the promotion of Oprah Winfrey, admits that he can't be completely vegetarian although his wife is. He goes on to say that he only eats meat once a week which is virtually vegetarian. He says that he has problems with beef sometimes.

Since I support a transition toward a diet based on mostly fresh, living fruits, vegetables and cultured milk products like yogurt and cheese, I support the flexitarian and Meatless Mondays campaigns.

I offer vegetarian recipes based on green leafy vegetables, tomato and cucumber and cooked starchy vegetables like broccoli, cauliflower, cabbage and squash beside potatoes and whole grains. I would take the recipes given by the Meatless Mondays and flexitarian movements, which are largely grain, bean and pasta based, and add a big green leafy salad and steamed vegetables to balance it out. As entrees the recipes are fine, but always remember to start a vegetable meal with a large green salad and steamed veggies, and then eat the grain, potato or pasta entree. Soy and other beans can be problematic due to their indigestibility and gas production unless fermented like in tempeh.

Meatless Monday was recreated in 2003 as a public health awareness program in association with Johns Hopkins Bloomberg School of Public Health's Center for a Livable Future. The campaign was endorsed by over 20 schools of public health. Its goal was to help Americans reduce their risk of preventable disease by cutting back saturated fat.

The idea itself had its beginnings during World War I, when the U.S. Food Administration urged families to reduce consumption of key staples to aid the war effort. "Food Will Win the War," the government proclaimed, and "Meatless Monday" and "Wheatless Wednesday" were introduced to encourage Americans to do their part.

Herbert Hoover was then head of the Food Administration and spearheaded implementation of the campaign. In addition to advertising, his office created and distributed recipe booklets and menus in newspapers, magazines and pamphlets.

The effect was overwhelming. Some 10 million families, 7,000 hotels and nearly 425,000 food dealers pledged to observe national meatless days. In November 1917, New York City hotels saved some 116 tons of meat over the course of just one week. According to a 1929 Saturday Evening Post article, "Americans began to look seriously into the question of what and how much they were eating. Lots of people discovered for the first time that they could eat less and feel no worse – frequently for the better." The campaign returned during World War II and beyond, when Presidents Franklin D. Roosevelt and Harry S. Truman used rationing to help feed war-ravaged Europe. So, to help win two wars Americans gave up meat. Now, we need to give up eating so much meat for our health, the climate problem, sustainability and to stop the abuse and killing animals on factory farms.

Strict vegans and vegetarians need to embrace this movement as a step in the right direction and not criticize it for being a non-purist, non-ideal form of veganism or vegetarianism. 2 out of 3 vegetarians sometimes fail to live up to their ideals, so even the purists fail to live strictly vegan or vegetarian.

On her Vegan Challenge episode Oprah teamed up with food experts Michael Pollan and Kathy Freston to encourage her viewers to make conscientious, healthful decisions about the food on their plates.

Activist and author Michael Pollan shared that "75% of healthcare spending is on chronic diseases associated with diet." He went on to praise initiatives that challenge Americans to think before they bite, saying "anything that makes us become more conscious about what we eat is the first step."

Oprah and 378 of her staff members highlighted the positive effects and wide array of options available with a plant-based diet. To further encourage healthy choices, Oprah enthusiastically instituted Meatless Mondays at Harpo studios.

Giving up meat on Monday is a great beginner's orientation to a meat-reduced or meat-free lifestyle. Most people go cold turkey into a vegan or vegetarian diet and that can be overwhelming. So, it's best to cut out meat one day a week to start so you can slowly transition to a reduced meat diet. Then, when you are ready, add another meat-free day.

You also could let go of red meat and eat chicken, turkey, cheese, eggs and tempeh. You can order vegetarian entrees at restaurants and buy packaged vegetarian dishes at the supermarket. Remember to eat a vegetable salad and steamed vegetables before your vegetarian entree based on pasta or grains to get the vegetable broom effect working. The vegetable fiber in salads and steamed vegetables will clean out the mucus and toxic matter in your intestine.

THE AGING PROCESS

TELOMERES AND THE SCIENCE OF AGING

The telomere deters the degradation of genes near the ends of chromosomes by allowing chromosome ends to shorten, which necessarily occurs during chromosome replication. Telomeres are disposable buffers at the ends of chromosomes which are consumed during cell division and are replenished by the enzyme telomerase.

As we age, due to each new cell division, the telomere ends are not completely replenished and become shorter which creates a loss of DNA in the new cell, making it not quite as good or older. If the telomeres are too short the cells cannot replicate and we die.

Elizabeth Blackburn PhD, professor of biochemistry and biophysics at UCSF in 1984 discovered that the enzyme telomerase has the ability to lengthen telomeres and thus allow cells to replicate without a loss of DNA which implies telomerase can reverse the aging of process at the cellular level.

This breakthrough discovery led to the 2009 Nobel Prize in physiology. Elizabeth along with Carol Greider and Jack Szostak were jointly awarded the Nobel Prize in Physiology or Medicine in 2009 "for the discovery of how chromosomes are protected by telomeres and the enzyme telomerase."

This is great news because short telomeres are a risk factor not just for death itself, but for many diseases as well. Telomere shortening has been linked to: decreased immune response against infections, type 2 diabetes, atherosclerotic lesions, neuro-degenerative diseases, testicular, splenic, intestinal atrophy and DNA damage.

If you could unravel the tip of the chromosome, a telomere is about 15,000 bases long at the moment of conception in the womb and 10,000 bases long at birth. Immediately after conception your cells begin to divide, and your telomeres shorten each time the cell divides.

Once your telomeres have been reduced to about 5,000 bases, you essentially die of old age.

Many studies have demonstrated links between chronic stress and indices of poor health, including risk factors for cardiovascular disease and poorer immune function. The exact mechanism, however, of how stress ruins your health remained unknown.

Blackburn and Epel investigated the hypothesis that stress impacts health by modulating the rate of cellular aging (Epel et al, 2004). Blackburn and Epel found irrefutable evidence that psychological stress, both perceived stress and continual, long-term stress, is significantly associated with higher oxidative stress, lower telomerase enzyme activity and shorter telomere length, which are known determinants of cell aging and longevity, in the lymphocytes (key cells of the immune system) of healthy premenopausal women.

Women with the highest levels of perceived stress have telomeres shorter on average by the equivalent of at least 10 years of additional aging compared to low stress women.

In a recent study (Puterman et al, 2010) exercise was shown to buffer the effects of stress on telomere length. Among the women who did not exercise, each unit increase in the Perceived Stress Scale was related to a 15-fold increase in the odds of having short telomeres. Those who did exercise regularly showed no correlation between telomere length and perceived stress. That's great news! Exercise can nullify the aging effects of stress. Stress and especially major stress events like a relative's death, can be treated with regular exercise.

In 2009 it was found that taking a multivitamin increases your telomere length (Xu Q et al, 2009). On average the women who took multivitamin supplements had five percent longer telomeres than women who took no supplements which means that their biological age was ten years younger. Supplements that only contain B-vitamins or stress reducers, have no effect on telomere length. Multivitamin preparations containing antioxidants were better than other types of multivitamins. The telomeres of the women who took antioxidant multivitamins were eight percent longer than normal.

Some women took supplements that only contained a few micronutrients. These had no effect. Pills containing only iron actually shorten the telomeres. Supplements with extra B12 were an exception. Vitamin B-12 lengthens the telomeres. Vitamins and minerals that increase telomere length are:
Folate; This B vitamin is important for DNA and RNA structure and function.
Vitamin B12; In conjunction with folate, this B vitamin is important for the methylation, or detoxification, of homocysteine. Higher levels of homocysteine are associated with increased oxidative stress.
Niacin (nicotinamide); Can influence telomere length through its

multiple regulatory and coenzymatic activities.

Vitamin A and beta-carotene; These antioxidants reduce concentrations of harmful signaling molecules and increase beneficial ones to help reduce oxidative stress.

Vitamin D; Higher levels of vitamin D lower levels of c-reactive protein (CRP), a protein with harmful effects and associated with shortened telomere length and inflammation. Vitamin D appears to inhibit some of CRP's harmful effects.

Vitamins C and E; These antioxidant vitamins are widely acknowledged for limiting oxidative stress and its damage on DNA and telomeres.

Magnesium; The mineral required for the activity of a number of enzymes involved in DNA replication and repair. Low amounts of this mineral are also associated with higher concentrations of CRP.

Zinc; This mineral is necessary for a variety of enzymes including DNA polymerases, which are important for DNA and telomere maintenance.

Iron; In contrast to the other nutrients, iron supplementation is associated with shorter telomeres. This is likely because of iron's pro-oxidant ability to stimulate free radical generation. While iron supplements may increase oxidative stress, iron from diet or multivitamins (containing less iron) is not negatively associated with telomere length.

Other Bioactives are:

Curcumin and turmeric – Turmeric, and its primary component curcumin, are common dietary spices that stimulate synthesis of antioxidants, thereby protecting against oxidative stress. Mice fed diets containing curcumin had a trend for longer telomeres compared with controls.

Long-chain omega-3 fatty acids; Higher plasma levels of long-chain omega-3 fatty acids docosahexaenoic acid (DHA) and eicosapentaenoic acid (EPA) may protect against oxidative stress by enhancing activity of the antioxidant enzymes superoxide dismutase, catalase, and glutathione peroxidase.

Polyphenols; Polyphenols from grape seed and green tea provide additional protection for DNA and telomeres from oxidative stress. Those who drink green tea regularly have longer telomeres while mice fed grape seed polyphenols had longer telomeres compared to controls. Dark grapes and blackberries are high in polyphenols.

Carnosine in one study (Preston, Hipkiss, Himsworth, Romero, & Abbott, 1998) showed it was the only antioxidant to significantly protect cellular chromosomes from oxidative damage. Other antioxidants cannot completely protect proteins.

Some of the age-related conditions that carnosine may help to prevent (and treat) include: neurological degeneration, cellular senescence (cell aging), cross-linking of the eye lens, accumulation of damaged proteins, muscle atrophy, brain circulatory deficit, cross-linking of skin collagen, LDL cholesterol oxidation, DNA chromosome damage and formation of advanced glycation end products (AGEs).

Carnosine is a dipeptide of the amino acids beta-alanine and histidine. Cheese is higher in protein than yogurt and would have a higher content of carnosine. Spirulina's amino acids help carnosine creation.

Beta-Alanine supplementation has been shown by two studies to increase the level of carnosine in the muscles (Harris et al, 2006), (Hill et al, 2007). The Harris study mentioned has shown that you can take an amount between 3.2 grams and 6.4 grams per day to significantly boost carnosine levels and improve performance.

Why not take carnosine directly and not beta-alanine? When you ingest the supplement carnosine, most of it is broken down in the gastrointestinal (GI) tract into beta-alanine and histidine. Some carnosine may escape the GI tract freely but is quickly broken down by the enzyme carnosinase. Beta-alanine and histidine are then taken into the muscle, where they are converted back into carnosine by the enzyme carnosine synthetase.

You would have to take substantially more carnosine just to approach the increased concentrations of carnosine achieved by taking the scientifically recommended dose of beta-alanine which is between 3.2 grams and 6.4 grams per day. It has been suggested that 4 grams of beta-alanine a day will reach the carnosine levels that 6.4 grams produce.

The dosage for beta-alanine used to reverse grey hair is 2 to 3 grams per day for at least 4 months to see results. During this time also take copper sebacate 22 mg and a good multi-vitamin formula. The multivitamin supplement will help boost thyroid function, which is essential to the production of hair pigment.

MITOCHONDRIA AND THE AGING PROCESS

The aging process involves a decreasing number of mitochondria per cell, which results in less energy per cell, because the mitochondria are the power plants of the cell. Mitochondria generate most of the cell's supply of adenosine triphosphate (ATP), which is used in the sodium/potassium pump to create electric potential differences which results in the creation of bioelectricity.

What happens as you age is that you end up with fewer and fewer mitochondria per cell and also a lot of the ones that still exist are damaged and not working so well. As you get older you feel like you have less energy because your mitochondria are dying out or damaged. These damaged mitochondria also leak a lot of free radicals. You can make new mitochondria through exercise, but there are other ways of doing it. Arginine in conjunction with choline and vitamin B-5 or pantothenate is able to make new mitochondria.

It just so happens that the best vitamins for men to take 45 minutes before having sex are arginine, choline and vitamin B-5. This provides more nitric oxide which is essential for an erection.

Physicians suggest that a standard dose of L-arginine in pill-form can be one to three grams with a maximum of nine grams in a 24-hour period. Another way to supplement your diet with this amino acid is eating arginine rich foods such as natural, grass-fed dairy products.

Food sources of Arginine (per 100 grams)

Mozzarella cheese, part skim milk	1042 mg (3.5 ounces)
Mozzarella cheese whole milk low moisture	928 mg
Mexican cheese, queso asadero similar to Monterrey Jack cheese	760 mg
Cottage Cheese, creamed, large or small curd	497 mg
Spirulina One tablespoon (7 grams)	290 mg
Yogurt, plain, whole milk	104 mg

The AI or Adequate Intake of choline for male adults; 19 years and older is 550 mg per day for men and 425 mg per day for women. Strict vegetarians who consume no milk or eggs may be at risk of inadequate choline intake. One cup of cooked, chopped broccoli has 62 mg of choline. Dried whey has 225 mg of choline per 100 grams or 3.5 ounces. Fruits including avocados, which is the highest fruit in choline, are poor sources of this nutrient. A whole small avocado (136 grams) has only 19.3 mg of choline.

So, what really causes the aging process? Dr. Denham Harman's Free Radical Theory of Aging and Age-Related Diseases, first presented in 1956, has held up very well over the years. In 1972 he extended the idea to implicate mitochondrial production of reactive oxygen species (ROS) such as H2O2 (hydrogen peroxide) and OH- (hydroxyl radical).

Dr. Harman realized quite early on that most antioxidants do not get into the mitochondria where the free radicals are generated and the most serious problem with free radicals is inside the mitochondria themselves. The only antioxidants that can get into the mitochondria are superoxide dismutase, coenzyme Q10, glutathione and catalase. Catalase is the most powerful of the mitochondrial antioxidants. Superoxide dismutase, catalase, and glutathione peroxidase decline with advancing age.

Glutathione cannot be taken as a supplement it must be made in the cell. N-Acetyl-Cysteine (NAC) acts as a precursor of glutathione. NAC is quickly metabolized into glutathione once it enters the body. It has been proven in numerous scientific studies and clinical trials to boost intracellular production of glutathione and is approved by the FDA for treatment of acetaminophen overdose. Because of glutathione's mucolytic action, NAC (brand name Mucomyst) is commonly used in the treatment of lung diseases like cystic fibrosis, bronchitis and asthma.

Alpha lipoic acid increases the levels of intra-cellular glutathione, and is a natural antioxidant, made by the body, with free radical scavenging abilities. It has the ability to regenerate oxidized antioxidants like Vitamin C and E and helps to make them more potent. ALA is also known for its ability to enhance glucose uptake and may help prevent the cellular damage accompanying the complications of diabetes. It also has a protective effect on the brain.

Selenium is a co-factor for the enzyme glutathione peroxidase. Selenium supplements have become popular because some studies suggest they may play a role in decreasing the risk of certain cancers, and in how the immune system and the thyroid gland function. However, too much selenium can cause some toxic effects including gastrointestinal upset, brittle nails, hair loss and mild nerve damage.

Coenzyme Q-10 (CoQ-10) is a vitamin-like substance found throughout the body, but especially in the heart, liver, kidney, and pancreas. Coenzyme Q-10 can also be made in the laboratory. Coenzyme Q-10 has a role in producing ATP, a molecule in body cells that functions like a rechargeable battery in the transfer of energy. Coenzyme Q-10 has been tried for treating inherited or acquired disorders that limit energy production in the cells of the body (mitochondrial disorders), and for improving exercise performance.

Ubiquinone is the fat soluble, oxidized form of CoQ-10. Ubiquinol is the reduced form and has far greater water solubility and much better absorption than ubiquinone. Healthy individuals under the age of 40 years, can effectively convert ubiquinone into ubiquinol. The ubiquinol form of CoQ-10 is the most effective for individuals 40 years and older or those at any age suffering with ill health. Absorption is a key factor with any supplement, including CoQ-10.

Carnosine increases catalase production which will reduce hydrogen peroxide levels. In addition carnosine also showed it was the only antioxidant to significantly protect cellular chromosomes from oxidative damage (Preston, Hipkiss, Himsworth, Romero, & Abbott, 1998). The best way to increase body carnosine levels is to take beta-alanine or increase your protein intake by eating more cheese and spirulina.

Dr. Bruce Ames and his co-researchers, found that in aged rats, lipoic acid and acetyl-L-carnitine significantly protected mitochondria from oxidative damage and age-associated decay (Liu, Atamna, Kuratsune, & Ames, 2002). According to the authors, "feeding old rats acetyl-L-carnitine plus lipoic acid restores mitochondrial function, lowers oxidants, improves the age-associated decline in ambulatory activity and memory and prevents mitochondria from oxidative decay and dysfunction."

Western biochemical science discovered these mysteries of the body's mitochondria. The greatest strength of Western medicine is it's mechanistic viewpoint, that is, a disease is caused by a mechanism or metabolic, step by step pathway. If you understand what those mechanisms are you can rationally design a process for intervening in those mechanisms to prevent the disease from causing damage and to eliminate the disease. The problem with the traditional medical systems like Ayurvedic medicine, Traditional Chinese Medicine and even Natural Hygiene is that they talk in more broad, general terms like "hot" and "cold." They are not based on specific biochemical mechanisms.

Another nutrient needed to extend human life is taurine, a sulfur-containing amino acid. It is very important for protecting electrically-active tissue like the heart, the eyes, and the brain. Taurine can be found in dairy products like cheese, cottage cheese and yogurt.

If you don't have enough B-6, B-12 and folic acid, homocysteine can build up which promotes atherosclerosis (the build-up of plaque in the arteries). Levels of homocysteine in the blood that are considered normal, are in fact atherogenic, and a risk factor for cardiovascular disease according to Durk Pearson and Sandy Shaw. Most people are simply not getting enough folic acid, B-6, and B-12 to prevent homocysteine caused atherosclerosis. If a person wants to get protective levels and to dramatically reduce their levels of homocysteine, one needs to take these water-soluble vitamins three or four times per day and at doses substantially more than recommended levels.

According to Durk Pearson and Sandy Shaw, the well-known life extension researchers, to increase your memory and cognitive performance (mental processes) take **choline** and a number of cofactors to maximize the conversion to acetylcholine:

1. Vitamin B-5 or calcium pantothenate (pantothenic acid) works through coenzyme A to increase the acetylation of the choline to form acetylcholine.

2. Another cofactor is **betaine,** also called **trimethylglycine (TMG)** since it spares choline from being transformed into other chemicals. A lot of the choline that you take gets oxidized into betaine, and by providing the betaine you can reduce that loss.

3. Another cofactor is **phenylalanine** which can be used to make the neuromodulator betaphenethylamine.

4. You also need vitamin **B-6** or **pyridoxine** which is necessary to form noradrenaline, dopamine, and betaphenethylamine and **copper** to help the reactions.

A United States government report from the Agency for Health care Research and Quality examined the literature on SAM-e (S-adenosylmethionine, a naturally occurring chemical found in every living cell) for treating three different conditions: depression, osteo-arthritis, and liver disease.

They found that prescription drugs were better for liver disease but for treating osteo-arthritis and depression SAM-e was quite effective and quite comparable to the prescription drugs. It works much faster in treating depression than Prozac.

HOW EXCESS FRUCTOSE CONSUMPTION
CAN LEAD TO DISEASE

Consuming excessive fructose can cause a number of serious health problems. Fructose, especially from soft drinks sweetened with high fructose corn syrup, sweetened fruit drinks and even fruit juices, ripe bananas and dried fruit, is turned into free fatty acids, very-low-density lipoprotein or VLDL (the damaging form of cholesterol) and triglycerides all of which get stored as fat. The fatty acids created during fructose metabolism accumulate as fat droplets in your liver and skeletal muscle tissues, causing insulin resistance and non-alcoholic fatty liver disease. Insulin resistance can progress to metabolic syndrome and type II diabetes.

The metabolism of fructose by your liver creates a long list of waste products and toxins, including a large amount of uric acid, which drives up blood pressure and causes gout. Fructose is the most lipophilic carbohydrate, in other words, fructose converts to activated glycerol (g-3-p), which is directly used to turn free fatty acids into triglycerides. The more (g-3-p) you have, the more fat you store.

Limiting your total fructose and sugar is very important for anti-aging and longevity. Excessive sugar or fructose intake (especially from dried fruits, dates) increases your insulin and leptin levels and decreases receptor sensitivity for both of these vital hormones, which increases your risk of type 2 diabetes and accelerates aging in general.

Glycation is the process in which sugar bonds with protein to form advanced glycation end products or AGEs. This process creates inflammation, which can activate your immune system. Macrophages are scavenger cells that are part of your immune defense system and as such they have special receptors for AGEs, aptly called RAGEs (think: raging inflammation). These RAGEs bind to the AGEs in your body and get rid of them. The problem is that this defensive process can also cause damage; the scar tissue inside your arteries created by this process is called plaque.

The journal Nutrients published a report (Luevano-Contreras & Chapman-Novakofski, 2010) on the impact of fructose on aging, "The data are supportive that endogenous AGEs are associated with declining organ functioning. As of today, restriction of dietary intake of AGEs and exercise has been shown to safely reduce circulating AGEs, with further reduction in oxidative stress and inflammatory markers. More research is needed to support these findings and to incorporate these into recommendations for the elderly population"

The study goes on to say, "In the last twenty years, there has been increased evidence that AGEs could be implicated in the development of chronic degenerative diseases of aging, such as cardiovascular disease, Alzheimer's disease and with complications of diabetes mellitus. Results of several studies in animal models and humans show that the restriction of dietary AGEs has positive effects on wound healing, insulin resistance and cardiovascular diseases. Recently, the effect of restriction in AGEs intake has been reported to increase the lifespan in animal models."

AGEs are also implicated in diabetes, macular degeneration, cataracts, and both weakening and stiffening of collagen in the body. Healthy collagen helps you to look young and keeps your blood vessels supple. When your collagen hardens and weakens, then you start to look older and your blood pressure starts to go up.

Garlic contains sulfur, which helps your body produce collagen. Garlic contains taurine and lipoid acid which support damaged collagen fibers. Make garlic a regular component of your meals. Tomatoes are rich in the antioxidant lycopene which inhibits collagenases. Cooked tomato has even more lycopene than in the raw form: Cooked tomatoes provide 7298 μg per cup, while raw tomatoes provide 4631μg per cup. Collagenases are enzymes that destroy collagen. Vitamin C is critical for collagen production in the skin. Guavas are very high in vitamin C; 228 mg per 3.5 ounce serving.

Cells excrete AGEs into the blood serum which are then eliminated by the kidneys. The kidneys can often be overloaded by all these AGEs. This overload can form a positive feedback loop until the kidneys fail. This is a common problem with diabetics who often have excessive AGEs due to excessive glucose in their blood. It is not uncommon for diabetics to suffer renal failure and require a kidney transplant due to excessive AGEs. If your uric acid is high or you have gout it would be wise to limit your fructose to 15 grams or less.

As a general rule, a diet of less than 10% of calories as fructose is ok for most people. Moderate fructose consumption of less than or equal to 50g/day or about 10% of calories has no deleterious effect on lipid and glucose control and less than or equal to 100g/day of fructose does not influence body weight (Rizkalla, 2010). This study states that there is no direct link between moderate dietary fructose intake and health risk markers. Most of the studies showing excessive lipogenesis and other adverse effects are in the range 15 to 20% of dietary calories from fructose.

Let's say you ate in one day: Papaya, raw, 1 small (4-1/2" long x 2-3/4" dia) (152g), Pineapple, raw, 1 slice (3-1/2" dia x 3/4" thick) (84g), Strawberries, raw, 10 medium (1-1/4" dia) (12g), Apples, raw, 1 medium (3" dia) (182g), Tomatoes, red, ripe, raw, 2 large whole (3" dia) (182g). This yields 29.5 grams of fructose according to nutritiondata.self.com's calculator. In a sample daily diet, that includes vegetables and yogurt, with a total of 1412 calories, this yields only 6% of the calories as fructose. This is well under 10%, so you could almost double the amount of fruit above and be ok, which would be 59 grams of fructose.

Also we should remember that in vegetables and fruits, fructose is mixed in with fiber, vitamins, minerals, enzymes, and beneficial phytonutrients, all which moderate the negative metabolic effects of fructose. The issue of dietary fructose and health is linked to the quantity consumed, which is the same issue for any macro- or micro nutrient.

Glycosylation is a good process in the body. Glycosylation is when the appropriate enzyme makes sure a sugar gets attached to exactly the right part of the protein (or fat). Glycosylated proteins are used to fend off disease and inhibit the development of Type II diabetes.

Glycation on the other hand is when sugars accidentally attach themselves to proteins without an enzyme's help and this can result in sugars being attached in all sorts of unpredictable ways. Glycation happens by accident and only when our blood sugar levels are high.

Glycation is reversible as soon as blood sugar levels drop with most of the sugars and proteins disengaging and no harm is done. The problem is if your blood sugar stays high, as happens with diabetics or pre-diabetics, the sugar-protein combo will result in the creation of an Advanced Glycation End-product (AGE). Glucose is the least reactive of all sugars and is the primary sugar in our blood-stream. Fructose on the other hand is ten times more reactive than glucose (McPherson, Shilton, & Walton, 1988).

AGE's are dangerous because they bond easily to each other and to other proteins in a process called cross-linking. AGE's cross-link the collagen which gives our arterial walls and our skin their elastic-ity resulting in hardening of the arteries and wrinkling and sagging of the skin. AGE's cause the oxidation of LDL cholesterol particles, mak-ing them much more likely to become trapped in arterial walls which leads to heart disease and stroke.

Our body can break down and dispose of glucose-produced AGE's although over time they accumulate in our organs and tissues and we age due to the excess AGE's accumulating. The problem is that AGE's made with fructose molecules are resistant to our disposal system. Not only they made at 10 times the rate, they cannot be disposed of.

When researchers start looking at the tangles of twisted proteins which accumulate in the neurons of Alzheimer's patients, they dis-cover AGEs in abundance. This is likely to be the reason why other researchers have picked up on the association between Alzheimer's (and other dementia) and high blood sugar.

When AGE's pile up in the lens, cornea and retina of the eye they result in cataracts and macular degeneration leading to blindness. When AGE's accumulate in the fine tubules of the kidneys it results in loss of kidney function.

Consuming soft drinks sweetened with HFCS (high fructose corn syrup is 55% fructose and 42% glucose) or even eating a lot of dried fruit like raisins gives us a big shot of fructose and a big and instan-taneous increase in AGE production. High fructose consumption also leads to an increase in insulin resistance. Over time insulin resistance makes our blood glucose level persistently elevated, which is a second major source of AGE's.

If your doctor suspects you of being diabetic, they will often test your HbA1c (or A1c for short) level. When doctors test to see if you are diabetic they measure the level of a glycated form of hemoglobin called HbA1c. A high HbA1c. level indicates that there are significant AGEs present which is a sure sign that your blood sugar is persistently too high.

Observational and controlled studies have linked fructose consumption to Type II Diabetes, heart disease, stroke, blindness, kidney disease and even Alzheimer's. AGE research has come a long way in the last decade and may provide a unifying mechanism which explains why the incidence of these diseases is exploding.

Most studies say that the fructose in fruit is not the problem but it could be if one eats a lot of raisins, dates, dried figs, watermelon and over-ripe bananas. Let's say you ate half a ten pound watermelon at one sitting. That would give you 75.9 grams of fructose in one large dose. That amount would spike your creation of harmful AGEs. If you ate 30 large bananas in one day you would be getting 198 grams of fructose. Even 15 large bananas is 99 grams and still high. If you ate a pound of deglet noor dates you would be consuming 88 grams of fructose. A pound of raisins eaten at one sitting gives you 133 grams of fructose. A pound of dried figs would give you 102 grams of fructose. Overeating dried fruit and high fructose fruits like banana and watermelon is as bad as drinking a lot of soft drinks. A 12 ounce can of cola has 22 grams of fructose.

Of the top ten fruits highest in both fructose and sucrose per 100 gram weight or 3.5 ounces, the first 7 are dried fruits. Raw fooders have long known that eating a lot of dried fruits ruins your teeth but they didn't know that they were also causing problems to their internal organs.

1. Dates, medjool Fructose: 32 grams Sucrose: 530 mg
2. Raisins, seedless Fructose: 30 grams Sucrose: 450 mg
3. Dates, deglet noor Fructose: 20 grams Sucrose: 24 grams
4. Figs, dried, uncooked Fructose: 23 grams Sucrose: 70 mg
5. Peaches, dried, sulfured, Fructose: 13.5 grams Sucrose: 15 grams
6. Apricots, dried, sulfured, Fructose: 12.5 grams Sucrose: 7.9 grams
7. Plums, dried (prunes), Fructose: 12.5 grams Sucrose: 150 mg
8. Blueberries, wild, heavy syrup, Fructose: 9.0 grams Sucrose: 10 mg
9. Blueberries, light syrup, Fructose: 8.4 grams Sucrose: 410 mg
10. Grapes, raw, Thompson seedless Fructose: 8.1 Sucrose: 150 mg
source: nutritiondata.self.com, nutrient search tool

TOTAL FRUCTOSE CONTENT OF FRUIT PER SERVING SIZE

The following categories are listed in order of **most to least** amount of total fructose:

Fruit Serving Size Fructose Total Fructose

Deglet date 1 cup chopped 28.8 grams 63.8 g
Raisins, seedless 1 cup 43.0 grams 43.7 g
Grapes, seedless 1 pound 36.4 grams 37.1 g
Fig, dried 1 cup 34.0 grams 34.1 g
Cantalope 1 medium fruit 10.3 grams 22.3 g
Watermelon 1/16th, 286 gm 9.6 grams 13.1 g
Apple 1 medium fruit 10.7 grams 12.6 g
Pear 1 medium fruit 11.1 grams 11.8 g
Banana 1 large 6.6 grams 9.9 g
Orange, Navel 1 fruit 3.2 grams 9.2 g
Nectarine 1 medium fruit 1.9 grams 8.8 g
Peach 1 small 2.0 grams 8.2 g
Medjool Date 1 date 7.7 grams 7.8 g
Cherry, sweet 1 cup w/pits 7.4 grams 7.6 g
Tangerine 1 medium fruit 2.1 grams 7.4 g
Strawberry, whole 1 cup 3.5 grams 4.2 g
Blackberry 1 cup 3.5 grams 3.6 g
Raspberry 1 cup 2.9 grams 3.2 g
Deglet Date 1 date 1.4 grams 3.1 g
Plum 1 2 1/8 inch diam. 2.0 grams 3.0 g
Avocado, Hass 1 fruit .109 grams .191 g

Total Fructose is the sum of fructose from sucrose and fructose.
source: Nutritiondata.self.com

In Britain the sugar content of apples has risen by up to 50 per cent over the last decade. New breeds of apple arriving on the shelves have been cross-bred to give a sweeter taste. Sweeter varieties such as Pink Lady, Braeburn and Fuji are increasingly popular among British consumers. Figures from the British Government's Food Standards Agency show that ten years ago apples such as Golden Delicious, Granny Smith and Cox's Orange Pippin contained 10-11 per cent sugar by weight. New research by the U.S. Department of Agriculture found that the typical modern apple now has a sugar content of up to 15 per cent or the equivalent of four teaspoons of sugar.

In conclusion excess fructose found in soft drinks and other high fructose corn syrup sweetened foods and also dried fruits or very sweet fruits like raisins, dates and bananas need to be restricted. It should be noted that although fructose has been singled out, polyunsaturated fatty acid lipid peroxidation produces AGEs about 23 times faster than the simple sugars do (Fu, et al., 1996).

STARCH

Laundry starch and cooking starch are both considered poisons by the National Poison Control Center in the United States. For cooking starch the symptoms listed are gastrointestinal problems like intestinal blockage and stomach area pain. For laundry starch (with very long-term exposure through skin contact): significantly decreased urine output (or none), jaundice (eyes become yellow), diarrhea, vomiting, convulsions, collapse, fever, low blood pressure, skin blisters, bluish skin, lips, or fingernails, flaking skin, yellow skin, coma, convulsions, drowsiness, twitching of the arms, hands, legs, or feet, twitching of the facial muscles. If the starch is inhaled, it may cause wheezing, rapid breathing, shallow breathing, and chest pain. If the starch contacts the eyes, it may cause redness, tearing, and burning.

Volkheimer rediscovered the Herbst effect which is starch found in the blood and urine right after ingesting raw corn starch or cooked starch in biscuits (Prokop, 1990). The term "persorption" has been coined for this interesting phenomenon and it means direct absorption through permeable tissues.

Volkheimer also found that mice fed raw starch aged at an abnormally fast rate, and when he dissected the starch-fed mice, he found a multitude of blocked arterioles in every organ, each of which caused the death of the cells that depended on the blood supplied by that arteriole.

Biscuits contain cooked starch so the effect also occurs eating other starches (even baked or well boiled); like cooked potatoes, white rice, brown rice, cassava, tapioca and cauliflower both cooked and raw. Carrots have some starch but mostly they have a sweet taste from their high natural sugar content.

Starchless green vegetables include lettuce, celery, spinach, kale, cabbage, dandelion and parsley. Starchless vegetable fruits are tomatoes, cucumbers and bell peppers.

MAJOR STRESS INCIDENTS ARE WHAT
DRAIN OUR BATTERIES AND AGE US QUICKLY

Extremely stressful incidents like the death of a loved one, being robbed, scammed or attacked, a lawsuit, a major family feud, fighting with your spouse or significant other, being fired from your job, all call on you to expend large amounts of energy in coping with the problem.

Add to this worry and anxiety and fear which releases the stress hormones cortisol and adrenaline which drain your kidney's vital energy reserves. Even the small incidents like your computer breaking down or an unexpectedly high water or electric bill take their toll on your body.

THE BENEFITS OF LIVING AT HIGH ALTITUDES

A study of 1150 men and women published in the Journal of Epidemiology and Community Health (Baibas N, Trichopoulou A, Voridis E, Trichopoulos D, 2005) showed that those living at altitudes above 3,000 feet in Greece had a longer life expectancy than those living closer to sea level.

Not only did they live longer, but their heart disease rate was almost half of their lower lying counterparts. Researchers believe that the adjustments the body makes for high altitude living may be beneficial for overall heart health.

When exercising at higher altitudes the body has to work harder which helps to strengthen the heart and improves stamina and endurance. The study concluded, "Increased physical activity from walking on rugged terrains under conditions of moderate hypoxia among the mountain residents could explain these findings."

INCREASE LONGEVITY SLEEPING
NO MORE THAN 7 HOURS PER NIGHT

An increased death rate has been associated with sleeping 8 hours or more. It's a common belief that 8 hours of sleep is needed for optimal health, yet a six-year study of more than 1.1 MILLION adults ages 30 to 102 has shown that people who get only 6 to 7 hours a night have a lower death rate. Individuals who sleep 8 hours or more, or less than 4 hours a night, were shown to have a significantly increased death rate compared to those who averaged 6 to 7 hours.

Researchers from the University of California, San Diego (UCSD) School of Medicine and the American Cancer Society collaborated on the study, which appeared in the February 15, 2002 issue of the Archives of General Psychiatry, a journal of the American Medical Association (Kripke, Garfinkel, Wingard, Klauber, Marler, 2002).

Although the data indicated the highest mortality rates with long-duration sleep, the study could not explain the causes or reasons for this association. First author Daniel F. Kripke, M.D., a UCSD professor of psychiatry who specializes in sleep research, said, "We don't know if long sleep periods lead to death. Additional studies are needed to determine if setting your alarm clock earlier will actually improve your health." But, he added "individuals who now average 6.5 hours of sleep a night, can be reassured that this is a safe amount of sleep. From a health standpoint, there is no reason to sleep longer."

The study, which addressed sleep issues as part of the Cancer Prevention Study II (CPSII) of the American Cancer Society, also indicated that participants who reported occasional bouts of insomnia did not have an increased mortality rate, but those individuals who took sleeping pills were more likely to die sooner. "Insomnia is not synonymous with short sleep," the authors said in the article. "Patients commonly complain of insomnia when their sleep durations are well within the range of people without sleep symptoms." They added that physicians believe most patient complaints about "insomnia" are actually related to depression, rather than a diagnosis of insomnia.

The best survival rates were found among those who slept 7 hours per night. The study showed that a group sleeping 8 hours were 12 percent more likely to die within the six-year period than those sleeping 7 hours, other factors being equal. Even those with as little as 5 hours sleep lived longer than participants with 8 hours or more per night.

Although the study was conducted from 1982-88, the results have not been available until recently due to the length of time required to input and analyze the vast amount and variety of data from the 1.1 million participants.

Last night my body started to feel weak and sluggish at around 9:30 so I went to bed. I woke up refreshed and my eyes opened wide naturally ready for the day. The key to sleeping well is listening to your body's signals as to when you should go to bed. Sometimes you need to go to sleep real early like 7 p.m. You may wake up during the night but just staying in bed, off your feet, with the lights out will give you the deep rest your body craves. Sometimes when you are really tired from too much exercise or too much traveling or shopping you will need to go to bed early and get up late so the body can recover. When a sick or injured person is recovering they need to sleep and rest as much as possible just like the fox does when he breaks his leg, he doesn't move until it's healed.

There is often the temptation to stay up late and over-ride your body's tiredness but I believe this stresses your body and ages you faster. Occasionally on Saturday night it's ok to stay up late, as long as you get your 7 hours of sleep. So, if you went to bed at 2 a.m. you would need to sleep until 9 a.m. to get your ideal 7 hours of sleep. I learned in Chinese medicine that sleeping before midnight is healthier because energy peaks for the liver from the hours of 1 a.m. to 3 a.m. and therefore it is important for the rejuvenation of the liver to be in a state of deep sleep before 1 a.m.

Going to sleep at 11 or 11:30 p.m. means getting up at 6 or 6:30 a.m. to get 7 hours of sleep. Or you can go to sleep at 12 midnight and get up at 7 a.m. although it is healthier to go to sleep before midnight. I personally tend to sleep soundly throughout the whole night without waking if I go to sleep later, like at 11 or 11:30 p.m.

HOW LIVING WATER
ENLIVENS YOU

Living water is alive because it contains living enzymes, the spark of life. Enzymes contain the spark of Life or 'chi', 'chee', 'ki' as the Chinese call it.

Chi is a form of bioelectric energy uniquely associated with living things. The Chinese have studied this bioelectric "chi" for 5,000 years and discovered that it ran in specific meridians or energy pathways in the body.

This dovetails with the Kirlian photos of the aura or bioelectric field of living, uncooked foods showing large, bright fields and that of cooked food showing dark small fields.

To be the most vital that you can possible be, eat foods fresh and raw because they have the most "chi" in them. To feel naturally high or euphoric we need to eat foods high in "chi" which is found in living water rich foods.

The fiber doesn't contain the life force or chi only the liquid portion of the fruit or vegetable, which is called "living water". The best source of this living water is naturally grown, fresh fruits. Fruits are 70%-98% living water. Fruits have a much higher content of living, bioactive enzymes by comparison than vegetables.

Aging is associated with the water content of the body. Infants have a water content as high as 77%, an elderly person may have only 45% and an adult has around 60%. The first 10 years of life shows the most dramatic decrease in water content. We are told by health experts to drink 8 glasses of water a day to stay hydrated. On a vegetarian transitional and on a frugivorous diet you are being hydrated by the living water in fresh vegetables and fruits and not dead, mineral laden water.

Inorganic minerals in tap and spring water are deposited in the body causing arthritis and artery hardening. Distilled and purified water can drain minerals from the body. The living water found in fruits, vegetables, 100% pure juice and coconut water is healthier than lifeless; tap (can contain chlorine, arsenic and other toxic chemicals), distilled, filtered, purified or mineral water. You can make an herbal tea with coconut water. Lemonade is best made with pure apple and lemon juice. If fasting it is best to make a laxative sen tea with purified or distilled water to avoid inorganic minerals and other pollutants.

HOW TO DO THE TRANSITION DIET:
THE BASIC PRINCIPLES

OUR DIET IS A HABIT
WE ADOPT AND ADAPT TO

Most people eat the same thing day after day like cereal and milk in the morning, a sandwich, chips and fruit for lunch and meat, rice and vegetables for dinner.

A vegetarian may eat fruit for breakfast, soup and salad for lunch and broccoli and rice for dinner. The same menu is eaten day after day without getting tired of it. It's also possible to eat just vegetables, fruits and cultured milk, prepared in many different ways, day after day without getting bored.

Many social interactions are centered around indulging in food such as the holiday meal Thanksgiving with its turkey, Easter with ham and Christmas with turkey or ham and the birthday party with cake and ice cream.

A whole new eating tradition needs to be developed not based on sensual delight, but rather on how the food develops your mind and body.

The Sardinian mountain folk have the most men over 100 years old because they eat plenty of homemade sheep's milk cheese and vegetables like zucchini, tomatoes, potatoes, eggplant and fava beans.

The American (and many western nations) diet is based on cooked meat, potatoes and rice, white bread, hamburgers, hot dogs, French fries, pizza, refined wheat pasta, pasteurized, grain-fed, growth hormone injected dairy products and not many fruits and vegetables.

This is why there is so much heart disease, cancer, diabetes, obesity, mental illness and social violence in our society. This SAD diet (Standard American Diet) has a lot of processed carbohydrates like high fructose corn syrup and white sugar which triggers insulin overdose and the formation of advanced glycation end-products (AGEs) which can lead to hardening and clogging of the arteries.

The SAD diet also has a lot of red meat protein, cooked starch and processed oils which when eaten which clog up the body's elastic tube system (blood and lymph vessels) with mucus and plaque. The transition diet supports the general health and well-being of the body and therefore the well-being of the emotions and mental faculties.

AFTER A WHILE OLD FOODS LOSE THEIR APPEAL AS YOUR BODY AND MIND GET CLEANER

Some people can't imagine giving up meat and meat based dishes and all the noodle, bean, potato and rice based dishes. After a while, as you get cleaned out and more sensitive, you feel what these foods do to you and you realize that it's better to feel good and eat our Nature given foods, than remain a slave to old food habits.

Cooking and the art of fine cuisine is really a clever way to make unhealthy foods such as meat, grains and beans palatable by dressing them with lavish sauces and spices.

We really don't question the way we were taught to eat. Our parents give us their way of eating as children and we really don't question it until we reach maturity at age 18-21. Our culture also imprints us with its customs of eating that have been handed down for centuries.

If we get really sick, it makes us question our habitual way of eating. At age 13 I got acne so severe that it affected me psychologically. I was embarrassed to show my face covered with acne and blackheads. I was desperate to find the cause of my scourge so I started reading and found out that nuts, chocolate and fried food increase acne or "zits".

So I cut out all chocolate, nuts and French fries religiously. It helped somewhat but not completely because I was still consuming pasteurized fluid milk, meat, bread, spaghetti and other mucus forming foods which were the cause. If I had changed my diet to a fruit, vegetable and cultured milk diet I could have prevented so much suffering.

In the normal mode of eating, elaborate cooking and washing of dishes takes so much time and creates so much waste from packaged foods and cans. This simple way of eating frees up so much time and energy which can be used to do what is really important in life. Remember to keep the transition creative with new recipes.

RECIPE IDEA: Ratatouille: One large eggplant (aubergine), half a small squash (Japanese kabocha has the best flavor), 3 zucchinis, 3 large diced tomatoes and one large onion sauteed in olive oil or coconut oil until soft. Cube vegetables, mix thoroughly with the sauteed onions and tomatoes, add dried oregano, herb salt, then steam until tender.

AN INVITATION TO THE TRANSITION

I invite you to get to know your physiology because it's your source of health and happiness. Health education liberates us from ignorance and blind obedience to drug-based, medical scientists and vegan, raw and cooked food promoters, who both keep true health a secret from us.

Medical science has become too hard and rigid and has lost the artistic, intuitive part of healing. It's become overly dependent on drugs to artificially alter biochemistry, which really causes a suppression of symptoms which return later more aggravated. Diet is the way to naturally balance the body's biochemistry. Health education on diet, exercise and stress management is the key to creating healthy and peaceful people.

The transition diet allows one to detoxify slowly and safely, enabling one to gradually adapt to a balanced vegetarian or semi-vegetarian diet based on vegetables and fruits without dire complications.

The transition diet allows people to return to their natural purity in body and mind, as it was in the beginning in the original paradise. There we lived on the juicy fruits and vegetables of the garden supplemented by the cultured milk of the grass grazing animals and on the pure, rarefied air, sunlight, cosmic and earth radiations that naturally surrounded us.

Our occupation was caring for the fruit and vegetable gardens which in turn provided air to breathe, aromatic fragrances, living water, fruit sugar, organic minerals and vitamins.

The ecology of paradise was a balanced way of life, creating no pollution nor climatic imbalance. It was a self-regenerating, living system providing all the food, air and water needed for a simple, child-like, natural life for humans and all creation.

ADVISORY WARNING FOR PEOPLE ON MEDICATION, DIABETICS OR THOSE WITH OTHER DISEASES

If you currently have a serious health problem consult with your health practitioner (nutritionally inclined) to see if you are well enough to make a major diet change.

If you are using medications that are life sustaining, to stop them would be fatal. If your doctor says it's okay to taper off from the drugs, then you need to go very, VERY slowly in detoxifying the body, because stored pharmaceuticals and toxic pesticides will be released into the blood stream as you detoxify.

Diabetics ought to consult with an integrative doctor to see if it's all right to do the transition diet based on cooked and raw vegetables, cooked brown rice, potatoes, rye crisp bread, whole grain bread, whole grain pasta and a minimum of raw and cooked fruit.

THE TRANSITION DIET IS LOW IN COST

Vegetables like lettuce, carrots and broccoli, which are staples of the transition diet, are low in cost. At farmer's markets you can find low priced, high quality organic produce and can often glean over-ripe fruit and vegetables at no cost. Brown rice and potatoes are low in cost if bought in 25-50 pound sacks.

Ideally one will have some land, rented or owned, to grow vegetables and fruits in order to harvest your own fresh produce. The surplus can be sold at local stores, restaurants and farmer's markets.

Slowly, as more people become vegetarians or part-time vegetarians and are growing more fruit trees and vegetable gardens the whole world will change. The ecology and climate will stabilize due to more trees being planted and less being cut down for meat production.

FINDING INEXPENSIVE ORGANIC FOOD SOURCES

A move toward natural organic foods, avoids harmful agrochemical nerve toxins that were originally developed as weapons for World

War II. Seek out farmer's markets and natural food stores which supply organic and naturally grown produce at an affordable price.

Growing your own in a backyard paradise garden is the most economical way to go.

SEEING LIFE AS A JOURNEY
OR TRANSITION, NOT A DESTINATION

Learn to enjoy the transition journey. Work to see the perfection of Life as it is and as it unfolds. Everything has a purpose and everything has a cause and it's all revealing the innate perfection of all things. It really is all working for good, even if at times life is so painful. Pain is the teacher.

Staying in the present moment, free of the past and the future, is vital to being in touch with the ever changing needs of your body. Listen to the body, because it's moved by the Spirit. There will be good days when you feel energetic as a child and bad days when you are congested or cleansing and feel dejected and depressed.

Can you remember when you were so anxious to buy something you wanted so bad, and then the disappointment and dis-illusion when you find out it didn't make you happy? Things don't make us truly happy, nor does accomplishing temporal goals, just being alive and living in the magnificent flow and process of Life is happiness enough, a miracle.

The material world is transient like the rainbow and will passaway. Ultimate Health and Happiness is Oneness with the unchanging, uncreated, immortal Spirit.

Walking, swimming, running, yoga and weight training and sports like soccer, tennis, football and basketball all help you keep young and fit.

Hot spring, Jacuzzi, Turkish and sauna baths all help the detox process. Singing lifts the spirit and removes mucus from the lungs.

EATING CAN MAKE YOU
FEEL GOOD EMOTIONALLY

Not eating can make you temporarily lose control of your emotions. This could be mislabeled as bipolar or manic-depressive syndrome, yet it's really a failure to eat on time and of the right foods, which will supply essential blood sugar and stop the elimination of toxic material.

A vegetable meal with protein, fat and cooked starch will really make you feel centered, grounded and unmovable like a rock. A fruit meal cannot do this in a person who has not gradually cleaned out their body.

There is a rhythmic schedule and routine to the meal times. You will begin to feel a little less centered or stable as soon as you start cleansing too much or are lacking blood sugar. This can occur from 3-6 hours from the time of the last meal.

A GRADUAL TRANSITION IS NEEDED
TO ADAPT YOUR MIND AND BODY
TO A NEW WAY OF EATING

A gradual, long term transition is needed in a major diet change to adapt not only your body but your mind and all its habits and desires. If you cold turkey give up all unhealthy foods you will shock your body and your habitual mind patterns.

These habit patterns will come back and cause you to binge on all your old food favorites out of nostalgia and longing.

That's why if you do it slowly you wean yourself off the old stuff, and you will see what effect it has on your energy and emotions and thus you will consciously and deliberately give it up over time rather than forcing yourself with sheer will power to give it up all at once.

DOING NOTHING DURING
TRANSITION LOW POINTS

It's best to do nothing during low points in the transition. When you feel really weak or depressed, don't take any actions, just take it easy and rest until you feel better.

When the emotions get out of control we should avoid making any decisions or getting in arguments. Wait till the low period passes because they all eventually do pass. This is where your faith will take you through the hard times.

GRADUALLY REDUCING
MUCUS FORMING FOODS

Over the years, one gradually eats less mucus forming foods. Remember that cooked vegetables like broccoli and cabbage are not mucus forming and therefore won't slow down the elimination rate. Cooked potato, rice, pasta and bread are mucus forming and therefore will slow down the rate you eliminate mucus and toxic matter from your body. Vegetables act as an intestinal broom.

When just starting the transition one starts eating cooked starch like brown rice twice a day after the vegetables, then after some time, it's eaten only once a day, then later no starchy grains, pasta, potatoes or bread are included, but always eating striving to eat two big meals a day (vegetable or fruit breakfasts are OK as needed).

After some years and when ready one can eat cooked and raw fruit first followed a few minutes later by a raw salad with a raw yo-gurt dressing and cooked vegetables for your meals.

Suggestions for the cooked fruit meals are steamed apple slices topped with cinnamon and either raw, natural honey or maple syrup, dates (raw or steamed), dried figs (soaked or steamed) and soaked raw prunes (helps bind acid). Raw carob powder can be mashed with banana to your desired consistency making a pudding, moist brownie or a dry bread.

Gradually, just raw fruit is eaten before the salad. Avoid too many citrus fruits which are highly cleansing.

Green oranges, unripe grapefruits and lemons contain very strong fruit acids that can permanently damage the enamel of your teeth, especially if one sucks on them using the front teeth.

Eating only raw fruit or even all raw before doing a gradual transition-detoxification can cause cavities and tooth loss due to excess acids being released too quickly which acidifies the blood and due to the lack of calcium and fat-soluble vitamin rich cultured milk products. Eating plenty of raw milk yogurt and natural cheese ensures the right mineral balance for your teeth. Protect your teeth by rinsing with baking soda right after a fruit meal. Avoid brushing after a fruit only meal because the enamel is softened by the fruit acids and can be brushed away by a toothbrush. Brush and floss them after a vegetable meal.

The final stage of the transition is reducing unsaturated fat consumption (avocado, olive oil and olives). At this stage a sweet, juicy raw fruit meal can be eaten for lunch and a salad with cooked vegetables for dinner. One can eat lighter steamed vegetables like broccoli, squash (kabocha, acorn), string beans and artichoke.

The fat is olive oil (extra virgin), olives (Kalamata or Spanish), sour cream, coconut oil and butter. A "gazpacho" vegetable fruit salad can be made with chopped tomatoes, grated cucumber, grated bell pepper, avocado, spirulina, lemon juice, onion and garlic.

Olives are good as a side dish since they tend to bind mucus, yet they can be fattening if over-eaten.

Avocado is easy to over-eat on, so it's best to measure out before the meal how much avocado you are going to eat and stick to that portion. Avocados can be deceptive, tasting good, yet high in the cancer and heart disease causing polyunsaturated fats.

Olive oil is a safer fat but even then it must be portion controlled to avoid mucus formation and body fat. Gradually, over the years, one will need less olive oil, olives and avocado (high in polyunsaturated fats) and will live comfortably on the many varieties of fruit and vegetables supplemented by cultured milk (sour cream, butter, cheese, cottage cheese and yogurt).

Supplemental herbs, minerals and vitamins are needed to heal the body from past errors and protect it from current pollution.

A CLEAN BODYMIND IS
YOUTHFUL AND ENERGETIC

If you are doing the transition correctly you ought to feel energetic and uplifted in spirit. A cheery, happy feeling ought to bubble up naturally, because your vital energy is unobstructed. Wrinkles on your face will be reduced if you are cleansing properly, giving you a more youthful appearance.

HOW LONG A TRANSITION?

Too short a transition would not be beneficial because too many toxins are released all at once, which overworks the eliminative organs, thereby depleting the inherent vitality of the body. A longer transition preserves your youth and vitality. Too long a transition is just riding fences, playing around in the dark.

The length of the transition depends on how long one has been eating conventionally. Professor Arnold Ehret took eight years to completely clean out his system, but don't worry, the main thing is to start feeling better right away by the gradual elimination of toxic material. It also depends if you want to transition to a semi-vegetarian diet using cooked and raw foods, a lacto-vegetarian diet using cooked and raw foods (which will take longer) or a lacto-vegetarian diet using mostly raw vegetables, fruits and cultured milk (which will take the longest).

THE VEGETABLE BROOM AND
SLOWING ELIMINATION

Cooked and raw vegetables, with their high fiber content, physically sweep the whole alimentary tract, ridding it of mucus and stored toxic matter from many years of dietary abuse.

There are many tiny folds in the small intestine and large intestine where mucus and undigested food particles can get trapped which will cause an obstruction of the flow of food through the digestive system.

The course fiber of raw vegetables like grated carrots, lettuce and cucumber and cooked vegetables like broccoli, cabbage, cauliflower and string beans will physically brush the sides of the intestine making them clean so the digested food can flow easily along the digestive tube.

Vegetables both raw and cooked will not slow down your elimination, they will just physically clean out the digestive tube system. In order to slow down your elimination when you become toxic it is necessary to eat cooked starch and also enough fat and protein. Brown rice and potatoes are mucus forming which allows a slowing of the removal of mucus and toxic material from the body.

If you feel real weak and jittery it's time to eat some cooked starch in the form of potatoes, brown rice, rye crisp bread or whole grain pasta which will slow down the elimination of toxic material from the body and you will feel better almost immediately. These are two very important points to remember.

RAW VEGETABLES ARE NEEDED
FOR ENZYMES AND AS
A VEGETABLE BROOM

Raw salad vegetables include lettuce, spinach (good for binding acidic mucus and toxic matter) and tomatoes. Carrots finely grated in the salad are delicious. Carrots have a little starch which helps make the meal more complex and thus slower to digest. Paper thin, sliced cucumbers are a nice addition.

Organic bottled or homemade raw sauerkraut helps keep the digestive tract alkaline by neutralizing toxins and adds flavor. The vegetable salad can be made of raw lettuce, spinach, grated carrot, tomato, sliced cucumber, bell pepper and dressed with olive oil, olives, sauerkraut and mayonnaise or raw yogurt. Eat steamed vegetables like cauliflower, cabbage and broccoli, after or with the salad.

Lunch is eaten around 12 p.m. (noon) and dinner at around 6 p.m., allowing about 6 hours between meals, which gives the body ample time to fast between meals and thus detoxify. Eat earlier (10:30) if you feel weak.

Pure, distilled water can be drunk in between meals or use a good, reverse osmosis purified bottled water. Add a little lemon and lime juice and a little natural sweetener like raw, natural honey or stevia. Or use glacier source mountain water with low dissolved solids if available.

Avoid lemonade and teas heavily sweetened by raw cane sugar or brown sugar because they will rot your teeth quickly. By drinking pure water you are helping your body flush out the toxins.

Speeding up and slowing down the elimination rate is the artistic key to the transition diet. One can slow down the elimination rate by using heavier, mucus forming foods or use fruit and fasting to speed it up, depending on how one feels.

Remember to enjoy yourself in the transition which means not cleansing too fast, which makes you unhappy and irritable. Remember that a lot of the transition depends on the individual and therefore you'll need to experiment to see what works for you.

Intuition and trusting your inner common sense as to what you really need to be happy in the moment is what makes this way of eating work. It's how the diet makes you feel and act that's important.

If you need to slow down your elimination to be a more kind, selfless and outgoing person, then do yourself and the people around you a service, by eating to live as a more helpful and happy person.

Fruit is used in small quantities or avoided when first starting out on the transition, because it stirs up too much mucus. Steamed or baked apple is the exception and can be eaten before or with the cooked vegetables. A vegetable or fruit breakfast can be eaten, if needed so you can work in the morning, but to aid the elimination process just take liquids in the morning.

AVOIDING TOO MUCH FRUIT
SLOWS THE ELIMINATION RATE

Eating only or mostly fruit for weeks or months on end, or too much juice or water fasting creates an imbalance that often can cause a binge into many old problem foods. Being impatient doesn't help your transition.

Fruit, like steamed apple topped with a little cinnamon and raw honey or real maple syrup, can be eaten right before or with the vegetable meal or try prunes (soaked), raisins, dried mango and dried figs. These fruits won't speed up your elimination and will give you that taste of something sweet.

SLOWING DOWN THE ELIMINATION

Remember that steamed cauliflower, broccoli and squash won't stop the elimination as well as mucus forming cooked brown rice and cooked potatoes.

Rye crisp cracker "bread" (Ryvita and Wasa are two better known brands) has a lot of fiber to help sweep out the digestive tract and it will also slow down your elimination.

Organic brown rice will slow down the elimination very effectively, and thus should be used by beginners and more advanced transitioners in moderate quantities without overeating, since it can cause an arthritis-like condition to develop creating pain in the joints, if eaten to excess.

COOKED STARCH HELPS SLOW DOWN THE ELIMINATION PROCESS AND STOP THE "JITTERS" THAT COMES FROM CLEANSING TOO FAST

Brown (whole) rice or potatoes are needed to stop a heavy elimination if you are just starting the transition. Brown rice has the bran fiber which acts as a vegetable broom unlike white rice which is sticky.

Potatoes are less acid forming than brown rice, but more mucus forming. They can be cooked fast by steaming thin slices, or they can be sliced in thin rounds and then baked, or cut in cubes and then boiled. Brown rice or potatoes should be eaten at the end of the meal to ease digestion, thereby not confusing the digestive organs.

Rye crisp bread is good for the transition because it mechanically sweeps the intestine clean of hardened mucus and can be used when you are traveling or are unable to cook.

Salt helps dissolve mucus and helps in starch digestion. Nori and dulse flakes, kelp granules, Wright's salt and herb salt (herbs blended with sea salt like Herbamare by A. Vogel) are the best ways of adding salt. Natural salt is needed to season the brown rice and potatoes. Keep salt to a minimum because if you over-salt your food your kidneys will protest by forming lines and dark bags under your eyes. Use the least amount of salt needed to make the food taste good.

THE STOP ELIMINATION DIET

If you are cleansing too fast and getting thin, depressed, unhappy, unsocial, faint when rising quickly, always tired, your face is drawn, you have trouble breathing or other similar experiences, then stop your elimination by eating more cooked starch, protein, fat and less raw salad vegetables and steamed vegetables.

Avoid all fruit because it speeds up elimination. Stay with enough vegetables to have enough fiber for good bowel function. Eat a few lettuce leaves, grated carrot and celery dressed with plenty of protein, like clabbered milk, raw cheese or mayonnaise, plus olive oil, avocado, olives and then a little steamed vegetables like kabocha squash and cauliflower, then plenty of baked whole grain pasta, brown rice, well toasted whole wheat bread and rye crisp bread with avocado spread.

You are emphasizing the mucus forming starches, protein and fat and de-emphasizing the vegetables both raw and cooked and avoiding all fruit. This will provide enough mucus to stop the overly rapid elimination of mucus and various poisons stored in the tissues from 15, 20, 30 or more years of wrong eating, medical drug use and stressful living.

Stay on this mucus-rich diet for only as long as it takes to get back to normal, because if you stay too long on this diet you will pendulum swing in the other direction and become overly mucus clogged and congested. There is always a balance point that needs to be found between too much elimination and too little.

Excess elimination can be set off by stressful circumstances like traveling and eating food you are not used to. Fasting when you are not ready for it can also set off an acute elimination episode. Eating too lightly for many days in a row can also speed up the elimination rate excessively.

To stop an excessive rate of elimination you need to add meals. Eat as many times daily as needed to feel good on this Stop Elimination Diet. The idea is to stop your excessive rate of elimination by adding more mucus forming foods and adding meals.

EMERGENCY RELIEF

If you get an emergency case of severe gas and painful bloating take the herbal laxative senna for immediate relief. Senna or cassia can clean out the bowels as effectively as an enema and is more convenient.

A laxative will completely empty the bowels about five hours after taking it. Overuse of enemas can create a weakening of the intestines until it is only possible to evacuate the bowels with an enema.

A professionally given colonic or a high enema (cleans the upper colon) is useful for beginners to remove encrusted hardened mucus (mucoid plaque) that forms on the walls of the colon from years of abuse.

RAW FOOD VERSUS
A TRANSITION USING COOKED FOOD

Raw food enthusiasts deny the need for the use of cooked foods transitionally. Fatty nuts, seeds, avocados and durians are all mucus forming. Combining sweet fruit with nuts and seeds, and eating raw starch creates fermentation. Bad combinations create acid, alcohol and gas, which slows down their elimination, creating a feeling of relief from the detoxification symptoms of anxiety, weakness and depression.

These foods will slow down your elimination, but unless one does a deliberate transition using cooked and raw vegetables, cooked starch, certain fats and proteins, combined with fasting, they will never detoxify and be truly mucusless by avoiding all mucus forming foods.

Raw foodists never can clean out their bodies and will always crave mucus forming, disease causing foods due to their avoiding doing a proper transition.

RAW DIETS DO NOT CLEANSE THE BODY

Eating a diet high in vegetables and fruits without a prior period of transition can be damaging to the vital organs because highly toxic substances like fermented mucus, pesticides and drugs, which are stored in the fat cells and the intercellular spaces, will be suddenly released, flooding the bloodstream, which can damage the eliminative organs and even cause death.

Overloaded, the body cannot cleanse itself, thus, slowing the rate of elimination, assists the body's natural cleansing process. By slowing the rate of elimination you save your body's vital energy.

PROTECTING YOUR TEETH

Your teeth are in danger if one eats just fruit for long periods. Fruit sugar in a toxic body creates acidic fermentation which eats away at the tooth enamel. A lack of mineral rich, green vegetables and cultured milk demineralizes the teeth. Too much fruit also demineralizes the teeth. Only eat a moderate amount of fruit so that excess fruit acids and sugar are avoided. Sucking on unripe citrus fruits, like green oranges, eats away at the front tooth enamel. Dried fruit, sugar, raw cane sugar, maple syrup and even honey cause tooth decay because their high sugar content drains minerals and breeds bacteria.

Cleaning the teeth after every meal by using baking soda, a mouthwash, brushing (but not right after eating fruit) and flossing prevents the formation of cavities. Rinse your teeth with dry baking soda after eating fruit to neutralize the fruit acids. Avoid exclusive fruit diets and unripe citrus and pineapple and always get the acids off the enamel by rinsing with water when not home.

LIQUIDS HELP THE
DETOXIFICATION PROCESS

To help the detoxification process drink liquids in the morning and when thirsty. Liquids flush out toxic matter from the body.

Use distilled or reverse osmosis purified water tinctured with lemon and a natural sweetener like honey to avoid inorganic minerals. Glacier source water is a good low dissolved mineral solids drink if available. Mineral rich, ground water from wells or springs contain dissolved minerals, which take weeks to remove from the body and can be felt causing the joints to ache.

Fresh made organic vegetable juice using a juicer is a naturally distilled, living water (celery, carrot, spinach, tomato, cucumber and parsley is a good mix). Bottled or canned heat processed juices (V-8 etc.) are also good because they have less of a cleansing effect due to their lack of enzymes.

Herb tea sweetened with stevia is an excellent, soothing drink. Fresh fruit juice like pineapple, apple and orange are also good drinks to include in the diet in moderate amounts, but only if you use ripe, non-acidic produce.

STRIVE FOR TWO MEALS A DAY:
LIQUIDS AS DESIRED

Two meals a day allows the body to detoxify easier. As soon as you are able, try drinking fruit juice, vegetable juice, herb tea and lemonade in the morning or at night, as many days per week as possible until you can finally adapt to two meals a day.

Someone starting from a conventional, non-vegetarian diet can eat in the morning another vegetable or fruit meal if they are having problems with **THE TWO MEAL A DAY PLAN.** If you feel jittery and unsatisfied with many negative emotions you are probably cleansing too fast. The solution is to add more fat, protein and mucus forming cooked starch to your meals, but without overdoing it. The meal must be big enough to satisfy your hunger, so you won't feel weak a short time after you eat.

IF YOU ARE LOSING WEIGHT TOO FAST

Excess weight loss can be reversed by eating plenty of brown rice and potatoes and adding extra mayonnaise, raw cheese, raw milk yogurt, olives and olive oil or avocado on the salads.

Don't be afraid to eat enough mucus forming food, so you don't lose weight. Find that balance point where you feel good energy wise and feel good about how you look. Increase the amount of food you eat at each meal to ensure that you are getting enough calories. You may have to temporarily increase the number of meals you have per day to three or more in order to slow down the elimination process.

TRANSITIONING FROM A MEAT DIET

Those who have eaten a meat diet all their lives will have a lot of uric acid in their body creating an acidic condition. A vegetarian's body is more alkaline. If you want to eliminate meat completely, first stop eating meat (beef, lamb, pork), then later chicken, turkey, duck and fish. Then use tempeh soy burgers and marinated tempeh patties for a while, then later change to raw milk yogurt, raw cheese, mayonnaise, green pea guacamole, mayonnaise and spirulina. See the section on protein for the recipes.

LETTING GO OF MEAT

Homemade mayonnaise, raw milk yogurt, raw cottage cheese, rennet-less raw cheese, avocados, and tempeh are great meat substitutes when just starting out. Tempeh meat patties are excellent meat protein substitutes. Some tempeh products are marinated and taste just like meat. Excessive use of soy could lead to the formation of goiter or thyroid disease due to iodine deficiency (soy binds iodine) so it's best to use tempeh in moderation. Whether you decide to reduce meat eating and become semi-vegetarian or eliminate meat eating and become lacto-vegetarian, you are taking steps toward better health.

Removing foods that cause excess mucus and toxicity eliminates meat, poultry, fish and shellfish (fish, shellfish and poultry can be used transitionally), white bread, white rice, oatmeal, beans, nuts, seeds, eggs (transitionally ok to use), margarine, white flour baked goods, colas, coffee, tea, alcohol, all non-organic or commercial fruits and vegetables and all junk food snacks (cookies, cakes, chips, candy bars).

THE TRANSITION DIET:
WHAT TO EAT
AND HOW TO EAT IT

WHAT IS HEALTHY TO EAT?

Broccoli and cauliflower are two of the best vegetables because of their excellent flavor, but only if cooked because they contain a lot of starch which needs to be broken down by heat into simple sugars for easy digestion. Raw cauliflower can cause indigestion, gas and bloating.

Eggplant (aubergine), winter squash, zucchini, kale, collards, cabbage (cut in quarters or eighths) and string beans steamed until soft are also excellent. Cruciferous vegetables like cabbage, cauliflower, broccoli, kale, Brussels sprouts and collards are eaten cooked to convert their starch into simple sugar and ease digestion during the transition.

Cooked vegetables help slow down the elimination of waste due to their ample fiber, which absorbs toxins and mechanically sweeps out the digestive tract (which is over 30 feet long), thus preventing damage to the organs which must process the excess toxins being eliminated.

These cooked vegetables are not mucus forming (cauliflower is slightly mucus forming) and will not slow down the rate of elimination as much as brown rice, potatoes, olive oil and mayonnaise which are mucus forming. Cooked vegetables can be eaten after or with the raw salad. Raw vegetables provide food enzymes which help digest the enzyme-deficient, cooked vegetables.

THE TRANSITION DIET SIMPLIFIED

1. RAW SALAD

2. STEAMED VEGETABLES: BROCCOLI, CAULIFLOWER, WINTER SQUASH, SUMMER SQUASH, EGGPLANT

3. COOKED STARCH: WHOLE GRAIN RICE, POTATOES, WHOLE GRAIN PASTA, RYE CRISP BREAD

4. DO A ONE DAY FAST: USE THE HERBAL LAXATIVE SEN, THEN SKIP BREAKFAST, LUNCH AND DINNER, DRINK FRUIT AND VEGETABLE JUICE, BREAK-FAST THE NEXT MORNING

In order to recover from illness, use the above basic steps. Dress the salads and vegetables with yogurt, cottage cheese and cheese. Aim for two vegetable meals per day fasting in the morning on juices or tea. Eat only vegetables and no fruits on those days when you are losing weight too fast or feeling weak and nervous.

GUIDELINE TRANSITION DIET
DAILY MENU

Each person is a unique individual with a unique past eating history and degree of mucus congestion, therefore each person will need to experiment and find the detailed, specifics as to what works for them. Remember this when using the following daily menu guideline for breakfast lunch and dinner. Remember to be flexible and have fun with it.

BREAKFAST

"THE NO BREAKFAST OR NO DINNER PLAN": Eating two large meals a day helps the body detoxify faster. You can either skip dinner or skip breakfast whichever is best for you. The morning is the ideal elimination and cleansing time. Fast on air, also known as a dry fast, until comfortable and then sip coconut water and vegetable juice. Vegetable juice can help neutralize toxins faster. The juice combination of carrot, tomato, spinach, celery and cucumber will neutralize toxins and help move the bowels.

If you are unable to work well if you fast in the morning, then eat some bottled applesauce, cooked apple (steamed or baked) and naturally dried fruits like prunes, raisins, mango, pineapple or banana. These cooked and dried fruits that won't speed up your elimination too much because they lack enzymes.

If you feel really weak and jittery, eat a salad with dressing, steamed vegetables and a cooked starch for breakfast to slow down the elimination. Gradually work toward taking only coconut water, watermelon juice, vegetable juice, soup or bottled vegetable or fruit juices in the morning during this beginning phase of the transition.

Packaged, heat-treated juice has less enzymes to speed up your elimination, so it's a good choice.

It's important to feel good so you can work well and can relate to people in a friendly healthy manner. If you are cleansing too fast you feel unstable, jittery, like little pins and needles are bothering you, making you irritable and anti-social. In order to slow down the elimination eat a big salad with fat and protein, plus cooked vegetables and cooked starch like brown rice and potatoes.

Always remember to be flexible and eat as many times as you need to feel good.

LUNCH
In Three Parts

1. SALAD: Lettuce (red leaf, bibb, oak leaf, romaine, iceberg; sliced by a knife or torn by hand to the size desired), spinach, grated carrot, sliced; tomatoes, cucumber, celery.

Dress with sauerkraut (organic bottled type or homemade raw sauerkraut) seasoned rice vinegar or apple cider vinegar and moderate amounts of natural olives (Greek Kalamata are excellent), olive oil and avocado.

Homemade raw sauerkraut can be made by taking raw cabbage and juicing it in a juicer. Take the juice and pulp and place in a covered glass jar and let it set out until ripened which is usually 2 to 3 days depending on the weather. It's a very beneficial, toxin neutralizing food.

For protein use raw milk yogurt. To make it take raw milk mixed with store bought yogurt, a half cup per gallon milk, heated to 110 degrees F then kept warm wrapped in a blanket or put in an ice chest for 24 hours.

Or use homemade egg mayonnaise. To make it crack two eggs in a blender then add very slowly a half pint of olive oil, which is one cup or 250 ml, while blending, add lemon, onion, salt to taste. The dressings will be described in detail later.

Recipe Idea: Try a Spinach and Lettuce Leaf Salad; make a dressing of olive oil, lemon juice or seasoned rice vinegar, raw mayonnaise or raw yogurt, chopped tomato, chopped fresh basil, chopped cilantro, crushed garlic. Eat spinach and lettuce leaves whole by hand, dipping them one by one in the dressing. Serve with olives.

2. COOKED STARCHY VEGETABLES: Steam, or place in a covered pan with a little water at the bottom, your choice of one or more of; cauliflower, cabbage cut in quarters, broccoli, asparagus, eggplant (aubergine), squash, string beans.

Cooking these vegetables with steam converts their starch into simple sugar. Cauliflower is slightly mucus forming, the others are not.

To steam buy a metal steamer device and place it in the bottom of a pot. Fill the pot with enough water to reach the bottom of the metal steamer. Bring water to boiling then cover with a lid and cook at low heat. When it's soft but not mushy it's done.

Apple slices can be steamed and topped with cinnamon and honey or maple syrup.

Recipe Idea: A Touch of Italy: Sliced eggplant or quartered cabbage steamed with sliced tomatoes, sliced onion, oregano, herb salt and olive oil makes a delicious pizza or lasagna-like, Italian flavored dish.

3. COOKED STARCHY FOODS: Brown rice is good for those just starting the transition. Brown rice is more acid forming than potato making it good for the acid saturated bodies of beginners.

Season with a little herb salt or natural whole sea salt and olive oil. Eating only twice a day helps detoxify the body quickly. Eating big meals with plenty of cooked vegetables and cooked starch, enables you to feel good eating only two times a day.

Whole grain pastas like lasagna, spaghetti etc. are good to slow down the elimination for long term meat eaters just starting the transition (meat eaters are more acidic).

Pasta and brown rice can be used interchangeably. Pasta is cooked by quickly boiling for a short time (5 minutes usually) to soften to the right firmness called al dente.

To give the pasta a dryer chewier texture it can be put in the oven at 250 degrees F for 45 minutes after boiling.

The pre-mucuslean diet has cooked starch at both meals, the mucuslean diet has reduced or no cooked starch. Cooked starchy food is a staple on the pre-mucuslean diet and an occasional use item on the mucuslean diet.

Beginners in the transition start with the pre-mucuslean diet, then when ready, advance to the mucuslean diet.

Potato can be eaten after brown rice has been eaten for awhile. Potato is more alkaline and mucus forming than brown rice, making it good for stopping your elimination.

Potato is more convenient to use because it cooks faster. Potato cut in one quarter to one half inch slices cut widthwise, can be cooked in 15 minutes by steaming. Potatoes can also be cut lengthwise in half inch slices or in the shape of French fries and baked until tender and golden brown, then seasoned with a little salt and olive oil.

For **DINNER** eat the same way as you did for lunch. Remember to keep it interesting by trying new recipes.

THE SALAD DRESSING:
THE FAT PORTION AND
THE PROTEIN PORTION

THE FAT PORTION: Virgin or extra virgin (meaning it's not chemically extracted) olive oil is the easiest fat to digest and the preferred fat for the transition. Sour cream can also be used or a full fat yogurt.

Use only enough fat as needed. If you have excess mucus in the throat after eating then reduce the quantity of fat used. Olive oil is a good overall dressing with some lemon juice added to your taste.

Sauerkraut juice is a healthy alternative to regular vinegar or one can use seasoned rice vinegar or apple cider vinegar according to your tastes.

Avocado is best used moderately (a moderate portion in proportion to salad vegetables) since it's mucus forming (stuffs up the nose after eating it) and hard on the liver if eaten to excess due to its high content of polyunsaturated fat.

Avocado can be mashed into guacamole (mixed with finely

chopped tomato, lemon juice, cilantro, garlic) and eaten with the salad as a dressing or just eat a spoonful with a meal to satisfy that craving for something creamy.

Olive oil and herb sea salt (sea salt mixed with powdered herbs) can be added while steaming the vegetables to give them extra flavor.

Whole olives bind toxic acid lodged in the body which makes them very useful for reducing the toxic load of the body during the transition. Greek Kalamata olives have an excellent flavor.

Just a few olives are needed to infuse the salad with that olive flavor. Mash them and remove the pit, then mix with the greens. Kalamata olives are not treated with ferrous gluconate which can give olives a strange metallic flavor.

THE PROTEIN PORTION: The recommended proteins for those who have been eating meat for a long time and want to reduce it or give it up are mayonnaise, raw yogurt and raw cheese due to their ease of digestion. The easier to digest protein of cheese, yogurt and mayonnaise is needed to get off heavy meat protein.

This is **"THE METHADONE METHOD"** that heroin addicts use to get off heroin; using a less addictive chemical, then slowly tapering off, thus avoiding extreme detoxification reactions. So begin to add mayonnaise, yogurt or cheese to your diet and slowly taper off from eating meat to make the change easier.

"THE MAYO PLAN": Blending raw egg with olive oil wraps the protein in oil, which helps disguise it as a fat. This makes it easier to digest and is therefore the recommended protein to start the transition if you have been eating meat. Mayonnaise is made with two chicken eggs (free range if possible) with one cup olive oil, which is 250 ml or a half pint, slowly added while blending in a blender. If you have a handheld blender this eases the process. Lemon juice, onion, garlic and salt can be added for flavor.

"THE YOGURT PLAN": Raw, natural yogurt is made using a commercial plain yogurt as the starter culture. Yogurt can be used by those objecting strongly to using eggs.

Raw, homemade yogurt and cottage cheese are good when first starting out because it helps neutralize toxins and helps nourish the intestinal tract bacteria.

Raw cheese is heavier than cultured raw milk because it's so concentrated in fat and protein, but can be used if raw milk is hard to find or is too expensive. If raw cheese is not available you can also use a natural pasteurized cheese as opposed to processed cheeses like Velveeta and Kraft singles.

It's best to use raw milk to make yogurt but the yogurt starter culture can be from pasteurized milk yogurt. Free range eggs are the best to make mayonnaise and a good quality refined olive oil. The refined, cooking type tends to make a better tasting mayonnaise.

To get extra protein and trace minerals use a high quality spirulina and add it to salads. Protein is eaten with a raw salad to ease digestion.

Find the protein source that is easiest to digest. If you have been a strict vegan the raw, homemade yogurt will provide Vitamin D, B-12 and calcium which you have been missing.

The amount of fat and protein you use is determined by the reaction of your body. If you begin spitting up mucus during or after eating your meal, then you need to reduce the quantity of fat and protein used.

Nuts, seeds, beans and peanuts are not good sources of protein and fat because they are too hard to digest. They contain enzyme and nutrient inhibitors, which can be reduced by soaking and or cooking, but even doing this they're too hard to digest. They are too high in phosphorus which drains calcium from your teeth. If you use fish and chicken also use cheese and yogurt to make sure you are getting enough calcium and the fat soluble vitamins K and D.

PROTEIN: HOW MUCH DO WE NEED
AND WHAT ARE THE BEST SOURCES

Good sources of protein are whole, raw milk homemade yogurt, cottage cheese, farmer's cheese and other cheeses. Spirulina and chlorella are also good sources of protein.

The proteins found in meat, fish and poultry, cooked at high temperatures during grilling or frying produce heterocyclic amines which have been linked to various cancers including those of the colon and breast. Uric acid is a very strong irritant on the sympathetic nerves which gives meat that stimulating effect after consumption.

Eating too much protein (rarely occurs unless one is a bodybuilder or weightlifter overdosing on protein) releases too much nitrogen into the blood which must be removed by the kidneys, damaging them in the process. Acidic high protein diets cause the body to use stored calcium to neutralize the acid, leading to a weakening of the teeth and bones.

A low protein diet can cause hypothyroidism, where the body does not produce enough thyroid hormone to keep the metabolism high. A common symptom of hypothyroidism is cold hands and feet. Dr. Raymond Peat says that when the metabolic rate is optimal, most adults who aren't completely sedentary should have around 130 to 150 grams of protein per day.

Four ounces of meat contains about 25 grams of protein, however some dairy products have even more protein than meat: four ounces of cheddar cheese has 28 grams of protein. Having four ounces of cheese three times a day would meet the low, basic requirement of around 75 to 80 grams of protein.

A quart of milk contains 31.4 grams of protein and a quart of whole milk yogurt has 34 grams protein. Drinking fluid milk is not as healthy as using the easily digested, fermented milk yogurt. Three quarts or liters a day of yogurt is a lot, so it's best to combine eating yogurt with cheese to get the optimal amount of protein on a lacto-vegetarian diet.

Eggs are too high in PUFA (poly unsaturated fatty acids; omega-3, omega-6 can cause heart disease). Low thyroid function can be caused by the excess consumption of tryptophan, methionine and cysteine found in muscle meats and liver.

STAGES OF THE TRANSITION

STAGES OF THE TRANSITION

To make the change to a lacto-vegetarian or semi-vegetarian diet as easy and painless as possible, it's best to go very slowly, taking small do-able steps. This way you won't be overwhelmed psychologically and physiologically.

Preparatory Stage

The Preparatory stage is for those who have eaten a normal, meat-based, omnivorous diet all their lives and have never eaten a strictly fleshless, vegetarian diet for long periods. If you are vegetarian or vegan just skip this stage. If you plan to do the flexible or semi-lacto-vegetarian diet then just reduce meat consumption slowly by one half.

First Step: Let Go of Red Meat

The first step in going vegetarian is to let go of beef, lamb and pork and in their place use organically raised, free range chicken and turkey, organic raw cheeses, free range eggs and low fat fish from known clean waters. It's safer to stay with known toxin-free sources of meat and fish.

Organic chicken may cost a little more, but it's better than worrying about getting cancer. After a few months or years, or however much time you need to make the next big change, you can slowly let go of poultry and fish. Be sure you know which fish are risky.

Fish to Avoid

Avoid all high mercury fish and shellfish: albacore tuna; steaks and canned albacore, (note: canned light tuna, which is listed later, has a moderate mercury content), Atlantic halibut, king mackerel, oysters (Gulf Coast), pike, sea bass, shark, swordfish, tilefish (golden snapper).

Avoid farmed salmon due to its high pollutant content: Some fish are high in PCBs or Polychlorinated biphenyls which are neurotoxic, hormone-disrupting chemicals banned in 1977 in the U.S. PCBs are persistent organic pollutants (POPs) that accumulate in animal fat. Most farmed salmon are raised on feed that includes ground-up fish and sometimes other animals, like cattle, thus their bodies collect POPs.

Other POPs found in fish include the organochlorine pesticide dieldrin (water pollution from agro-chemical based agri-business) and dioxins which result from chlorine paper bleaching and manufacturing and incineration of PVC plastic.

Fish to Eat

Low mercury and Low POPs: Anchovies, Arctic char, crawfish, Pacific flounder, herring, king crab, sand dabs, scallops, Pacific sole, tilapia, wild Alaska and Pacific salmon (fresh or canned), farmed catfish, clams, striped bass and sturgeon. Children and pregnant or nursing women can safely eat the fish listed above two to three times a week.

To avoid excess polyunsaturated fat choose very low fat fish (less than 2.5 percent fat for each 3-oz. serving). According to the New York Seafood Council very low fat fish include clams, cod, cusk, blue crab, dungeness crab, flounder, grouper, haddock, halibut, monkfish, mahi-mahi, northern lobster, ocean perch, ocean pout, perch (freshwater), perch (northern), pike (walleye), pollock (Atlantic), red snapper, scallops, shrimp, snow crab, sole, squid, tuna (skipjack), tuna (yellowfin) and whiting. Clams, sole and flounder are both low mercury and very low fat.

Low fat fish will have less than 5 percent fat and more than 2.5 percent fat for each 3-oz. serving. Low-fat fish include bass, striped bass, catfish, mullet, rainbow trout, swordfish, pink salmon, chum salmon, shark, smelt and striped bass. Striped bass is both low fat and low mercury.

Atlantic cod, Atlantic flounder, Atlantic sole, Chilean sea bass, monkfish, orange roughy, shrimp and snapper are low-mercury but they are overfished or destructively harvested and as such should be avoided for the environment's sake.

Moderate mercury: If you can't find alternatives, then eat from this group, but be forewarned that the heavy metal mercury will accumulate in your body and is hard to remove: Alaskan halibut, black cod, blue (Gulf Coast) crab, cod, Dungeness crab, eastern oysters, mahi-mahi, blue mussels, pollack, tuna (canned light). Pregnant or nursing women and children can eat no more than one selection from this list, once a month.

Before eating fish from local waters it's best to check with your state's department of health for contaminant advisories. Avoid eating the skin and fatty parts of fish because that's where POPs collect. Avoid excess fat by eating baked, grilled and broiled fish but not fried fish.

Gradually you can replace the fish with delicious, seasoned tempeh patties, that compete with beef burgers in taste. For instance, you could try not eating poultry or fish one day a week and substitute it with a tempeh meat substitute.

Then gradually try two, three or more days per week eating a tempeh meat substitute, remembering that slow changes make it easier for your body and your mind to adapt.

Uric acid, pesticides, hormones and antibiotics are being released as you let go of meat, so you don't want to overload your bloodstream with too much all at once.

Brown rice and whole grain pasta is recommended during this stage of giving up or reducing meat, because they are more acidic than potatoes. This will help you come off an acidic, heavy meat diet because the grains will provide the acidity that the meat was formerly providing.

Eat a big lettuce salad and steamed starchy vegetables (broccoli, cauliflower, cabbage etc.) at both meals along with the poultry, fish or tempeh. The vegetables will help absorb the toxins that are being eliminated, as you let go of meat. Cooked cauliflower seasoned with lemon juice and herb salt tastes like fish.

The above steps also apply if you want to reduce your meat consumption, but not give it up entirely.

Pre-Mucuslean Stage
The next step, or the first step if you are already vegetarian or vegan, is the Pre-Mucuslean stage. At this stage you eat vegetables twice a day; salad and cooked starchy vegetables dressed with mayonnaise or dairy products, followed by a cooked starch like brown rice, whole grain pasta, rye crisp bread, toasted whole wheat bread or potatoes.

Use the more acidic brown rice, pasta and bread to begin with, then later use the more alkaline potato. At this stage you are eating protein, fat and cooked starch at both meals. The Pre-Mucuslean stage is a preparation to the Mucuslean stage, where the mucus forming cooked starches like potato and brown rice are slowly reduced. This stage can take a while, so take your time and enjoy the transition.

Mucuslean Stage

In the Mucuslean stage you are reducing the mucus forming cooked starchy foods like brown rice, potatoes and bread until you are eating no cooked starch. What makes this stage different from the Pre-Mucuslean Stage is that you are eliminating cooked starch (brown rice, whole grain pasta, potatoes, rye crisp bread, toasted whole grain bread) at one or both meals, until you are eating only salad and cooked starchy vegetables. At this stage you begin to eat small portions of cooked and raw fruit before the vegetable meals.

The salad is dressed with raw, made at home yogurt, cottage cheese, cheese and sour cream or egg mayonnaise. Raw cheese or a good natural cheese can be found at the market, since it's difficult to make at home.

In the end you are eating only cultured milk (cheese, cottage cheese, yogurt) or mayonnaise as your protein source and no cooked starch. Vegetable meals consist of a lettuce salads and cooked vegetables dishes like ratatouille and Bieler's broth soup besides steamed broccoli, asparagus and string beans. Cooked vegetables can help dress the raw salads. Some cooked foods like Bieler's soup you may not want to give up since they are so tasty and healthy too.

Mucusless, High Living Food Stage

In this stage you eat fruit only meals (different fruits can be eaten sequentially one after the other to prevent indigestion) followed by, after a 15 minute break, a vegetable meal like salad, soup or sandwiches.

Protein and fat sources are grass-fed, raw: homemade yogurt, cottage cheese, sour cream, butter and cheese (raw or natural).

Sweet, juicy fruit like apple and mango are eaten sequentially one after the other. Start with the most juicy, sweet fruit, like watermelon and eat it as a mono or one fruit meal and then follow with more solid fruits like plums and apples.

Allow a little time when eating melons to aid digestion (5-10 minutes or so) then follow with the next fruit. This waiting is important when eating melons, which due to their watery nature need to be eaten first and then take a pause before eating more solid fruits like apples. If you eat dates eat them last since they are dryer and more difficult to digest.

Make sure you eat within a one hour total time period for both fruits and vegetables to ease digestion.

Tooth decay can occur eating fruit only without vegetables or cultured milk or eating too many unripe fruit (citrus, pineapple, mango) and too many dates. Eat or drink only ripe citrus in moderation and juice or eat only ripe, sweet smelling pineapple in moderation.

Sub-acid, sweet juicy fruit like plums, peaches, apricots, apples, mangos, papayas, cherimoyas and all the many varieties of berries, grown on fertile, mineral-rich soil, preferable from your own garden, are the ideal fruits to eat.

Vegetable soup is a delicious way to drink your vegetables without the need for a fatty dressing. Juice celery, spinach, tomatoes, parsley, beet and a little cucumber. Filter twice, the third time grate 3 cloves of garlic into the sieve. Heat the soup so it's hot to the touch, but not scalding, this will prevent enzyme loss.

Burrito wraps of lettuce or cabbage leaves stuffed with; spinach, chopped celery, tomato and raw grated cheese or cottage cheese make a nice fast food alternative to a salad.

KNOWING WHEN TO STOP

At one point you will no longer tolerate very much cooked starch in the form cooked pasta, rice, potato, crispbread or whole grain toasted bread.

If you get violent gas, indigestion and skin rashes or eruptions from any of the above starchy foods, this is when you know when to stop. It's time to give up some starch and move into the mucuslean or mucusless stage when you get the signal.

Now this doesn't mean you will never eat starch again because if you have an elimination crisis you might need starch to suppress it temporarily. You also may hit another layer of toxicity at a deeper level and may need starch again.

But for all intents and purposes you are done with the starch, in the form of cooked grains and potatoes for the moment and can eat salads and mucusless steamed vegetables like broccoli, squash and string beans, cultured milk products and fruit. Spinach juice is laxative and can be combined with carrot, celery, parsley and lettuce to create a nourishing drink.

You are now entering the MUCUSLEAN AND MUCUSLESS stages but remember you may need to slow down in an emergency your elimination with foods like steamed cauliflower. In terms of the strength of mucus forming qualities the order goes as the following; whole wheat pasta is more mucus forming than potato which is more mucus forming than brown rice which is more mucus forming than rye crisp bread which is more mucus forming than cauliflower.

How much to eat is really guided by that inner appetite message system. That still, small voice that says that's enough. Watching TV while eating can interfere with this mechanism.

Eating really is communion with the Divine forces of Nature as contained in enzyme, vitamin and mineral rich living foods.

Somehow we lost the simplicity of eating. We fell into the habit of grinding the hard, dry wheat berry into flour and then baking it in wood or gas burning ovens. And later people sprouted wheat bread and then cooked it in the sun but this was also not our diet of fruits, vegetables and cultured milk products. Every meal can be a communion with the Divine as it was in the original paradise garden of fruit trees.

Eating for entertainment, like eating and watching sports programs or movies is losing the communal spiritual act of eating. Doing one thing at a time is an art, a meditation, while multi-tasking can cause loss of one-pointed concentration and the resulting stress and strain. Listening to the inner voice of moderation is practicing awareness.

Desire for more and being greedy and gluttonous really comes from not being aware, attentive, concentrated, residing in your heart, your inner spiritual essence. From the practice of conscious eating we become more aware in all our other activities as a bonus.

Eat enough so you won't lose weight or get hungry too quickly, but not to excess so you feel really bloated and your stomach aches. Enjoy your meals by making them a love feast. Try reclining in bed with your head propped up by a pillow on your back, completely relaxing as you enjoy every bite chewing it slowly, then when you return to the table you will be more conscious about eating.

Fall in love with eating again. Eating is communion with God, a love communion, a pleasure feast.

HOW MUCH TO EAT AND WHEN, IN ORDER TO AVOID DIGESTION PROBLEMS

THE IMPORTANCE OF EATING
AT REGULAR MEAL TIMES

Eating on time, at regular mealtimes, is very important to feel good on the diet and to maintain the two meals a day goal. If you wait too long to eat you get the "jitters" (irritable, weak, pins and needles).

11 a.m. or 12 noon depending on your work schedule and how you are feeling, is the time to eat a vegetable lunch and at 5 or 6, depending on your work schedule and how you're feeling, eat another meal.

If needed you can eat fruit in the morning until you can adapt to taking just juice or other drink in the morning. Or you may prefer to eat a large breakfast in order to work well and eat lighter or just take liquids at night. You can eat a little fruit (apple; raw or steamed, raisins, dates) with or right before the meals. This way you are eating sweet fruit without speeding up the elimination rate.

If you can comfortably go 5 to 7 hours between the vegetable meals you are making good progress in cleaning out your body. If you can go only 3 hours after lunch, then eat a more complex meal including more cooked starch (brown rice, potato, pasta, rye crisp), olives, olive oil, protein and steamed vegetables like cauliflower.

When first starting out, at every vegetable meal you are eating some protein in the form of mayonnaise or cultured milk and fat in the form of olive oil or avocado. Starch is eaten last to aid digestion. This avoids mixing starch and protein which can create indigestion.

Food will move through the body in sections or layers if eaten one after another. The order goes protein/salad first, then steamed vegetables; broccoli, squash etc., then cooked starch; brown rice, potatoes, rye crisp etc. Brown rice eaten to excess is acid forming and can cause an arthritis like complex to develop, so use it in moderation.

If one feels extremely weak waking up, then eat upon rising in the morning a salad dressed with protein and fat, cooked starchy vegetables and cooked starch for balancing. Then, when you feel better, try fruit in the morning and later just juices.

The goal is to fast on liquids in the morning because this is the time the body does its best housecleaning.

This whole process is **MUCUS MANAGEMENT: CONTROLLING THE RATE OF MUCUS ELIMINATION.**

The peak or highest energy periods of the day are in the early morning and right after eating lunch or dinner. Low energy periods coincide with when you start to get hungry; late morning and late afternoon. Not snacking between meals will free up a lot of energy that went into digesting food.

EAT TOO MUCH AND YOU OVERLOAD
AND CLOG THE SYSTEM, EAT TOO LITTLE
AND YOU DETOXIFY TOO FAST

Eat just enough food, but no more, to have a bowel movement right after eating. If you eat too much cooked starch, protein and fat, it will clog your tubes and cause sluggishness and lethargy. If you under eat on cooked starch (rice, potato), protein and fat you will detoxify too quickly.

Slowly, meditatively, chewing your food well is the best way to maximize digestion and also develop awareness of being full. Horace Fletcher was an American health teacher who recommended chewing your food many times until it's liquefied. He cured many people just using this technique because the food was liquefied and pre-digested which caused less clogging of the system.

Yet, he was not completely successful because the bread he liquefied still created mucus and constipation in the intestine, which ultimately brought about his demise.

As one gets more and more clean one gets highly sensitized to even the smallest infraction of healthy eating, whether eating too much rice or protein, or eating too many times, or eating something contaminated with pesticides or artificial fertilizers.

One can get severe headaches or gas and bloating. Eating a meal and then not waiting long enough to eat again can upset the whole digestive system causing gas and bloating.

It's best to eat again after 5 to 6 hours when the stomach is empty. It's better to eat two (or three, if needed) large meals than eat many smaller meals during the day because this allows the body to detoxify and rest.

WATCHING PORTION SIZES

Watch your portion sizes carefully especially of brown (whole grain) rice or potato so you can control the speed of your elimination. Eat too much brown rice or potato and you become dense and constipated, eat too little and you become irritable and weakened. It's a fine art to find that sweet spot in between the extremes.

THE BALANCE POINT: FINDING THE GOLDEN MEAN

The balance point is finding the sweet spot of moderation; not too much and not too little. Remember, if you are losing weight too fast, or feeling weak and nervous, stop eating fruit and just eat salad (with a dressing of protein and fat), cooked vegetables and cooked starch to slow down the elimination. Eat too little mucus forming foods and too much fruit and you start detoxifying too fast which results in irritability, weakness and weight loss.

Eating too much mucus forming whole grain pasta, brown rice, protein and fatty foods, will clog you up too much, eat too little and you will release too quickly your inner toxicity. Watch any mucus coming from the nose or in the throat as a signal that you can use less mucus forming foods.

Portion size is very important, watching that you don't eat too much salad, protein, fat, cooked vegetable and especially whole grain pasta, rye crisp, brown rice and potato, because any overload will slow down and bog down the whole system.

Both overeating and under eating creates a net obstruction of the organs which causes weakness and lethargy. As time goes by you gradually reduce the amount of mucus forming starchy, protein and fatty foods you eat, so you subsist on less and less.

The more mucus forming cooked starch you need to feel good, the more toxic you are.

You might ask, "Why can't I just quit all these foods and eat fruits and vegetables?" The answer is that for 15, 20 or even 25 years or more you have been eating wrong, so your body is saturated with waste products stuffed in deep layers within the cellular tissues that literally take years to remove.

NUTS, SEEDS, AVOCADOS AND GREEN PEAS

If one gets attached to nuts, seeds and avocados, even though they are eating all raw foods, they will never get free of their toxicity. Raw or not these concentrated fatty and protein foods will obstruct the flow of your energy and prevent you from completely cleansing.

The high polyunsaturated fat content is the problem with nuts and seeds. Excess polyunsaturated fat creates free radicals and robs oxygen from the body. The fat in sweet fruit, green vegetables and cultured milk is low in concentration and does not cause these problems.

Nuts and other seeds are not natural to eat since their purpose is to reproduce their kind, yet fresh, green peas are the exception to this rule.

Nuts and seeds contain anti-nutrients preventing their digestion as a defense against being eaten. Nuts and seeds give one indigestion and constipation.

Nuts and seeds even soaked can clog up the lymph system causing a sore throat. To trick Nature by soaking them to remove the anti-nutrients, fools no one because they are still too high in phosphorus and polyunsaturated fat.

Green peas are low in fat having just .22% by weight, whereas the almond is 51% fat by weight and is also 21% protein compared to the green pea's 5.4% protein. The popular walnut contains a whopping 65% fat and also is 15% protein. Cashews are 44% fat and 18% protein by weight.

Fresh green peas, lightly boiled or steamed or even eaten raw, digest well and are not constipating nor mucus forming if not overeaten.

The green pea is a legume but if harvested slightly immature, be fore it becomes hard and starchy, it has a green vegetable fruit quality rather than a seed quality. Fresh green peas are the best quality if grown in your own backyard garden using no chemical fertilizers or pesticides. Homegrown, naturally grown produce takes on a whole different quality.

The taste is like night and day compared to the mass produced green peas sold in the markets or in cans. A plant fed chemical fertilizer takes on a chemical, artificial quality that a detoxified person can see, smell and taste. If you can't grow your own green peas then go to the local farmer's market and look for the small scale organic gardener not the giant agri-business organic farmer. The small size gardener will have the higher quality produce. During winter if you are unable to find fresh green peas you can buy organically grown, canned green peas.

EATING LATE AT NIGHT
DOESN'T ALLOW THE BODY TO REST

If you eat late at night then you will be digesting all night long and will not allow the body to rest and recuperate. The nightly rest is very important and must be done fasting with an empty stomach. Eating dinner early and taking only filtered liquids if needed until the next day will allow the body to rejuvenate by fasting every night. Fasting is the key to health because the body rejuvenates itself by a complete rest from all digestion and activity. When the fox breaks his leg he instinctively knows to lie down and immobilize his broken limb and fast.

STAYING REGULAR,
FREE FROM CONSTIPATION

To be free of constipation one needs to find which foods are constipating and which are not constipating. Papaya is very laxative but eating a lot of bananas alone can be constipating. Yogurt and cottage cheese are not constipating but pressed, aged cheese can be constipating.

We need to experiment in our own bodies to see which food constipates our own particular body. Eating too early in the morning or too late at night can stop up the intestines. Eating too many times a day or eating too much in a meal has the same effect.

A natural rhythm must be arrived at as to when one eats and how much. Coconut water, watermelon juice and vegetable juice can substitute for a meal when you feel you need something to eat. For a pick me up when it's late at night or too early in the morning, try coconut water or filtered vegetable juice to prevent getting stopped up with constipation. Filtered juice is needed because the excess pulp in the juice can cause indigestion.

When it's really needed, like when one gets severe gas, fermentation, indigestion or constipation, take the herbal laxative senna. Herb teas containing senna can be purchased or better yet use senna in the bulk form.

Senna is useful when starting a fast to clean out the intestines which makes fasting easier since there are no toxins re-entering the blood stream from old feces in the colon. The short 40 hour fast helps clean out the intestine enabling good elimination and digestion.

In emergencies an enema can be used to immediately empty the colon giving relief from pain. An enema bag can be purchased inexpensively at a drug store and filled with warm water then inserted in the anus while lying down. The water is held until it is impossible to hold anymore. This cleans out the lower bowel.

A colonic will clean out the upper colon and can be used when first starting out on the transition to clean out the hardened black mucus clinging to the walls of the colon.

Keeping the intestines unconstipated and moving is very important in keeping the bloodstream clean. A backed-up intestine causes pain, bloating, gas and headaches, all the symptoms of IBS or irritable bowel syndrome.

What helps avoid constipation is avoiding constipating foods, overeating, too many combinations, too many meals and erratic meal times versus regular clockwork meal times.

THE CENTER OF YOUR WORLD

The center of your world is your abdominal cavity. It includes the colon, small intestines, stomach, spleen, liver and gall bladder. The roof of this cavity is the diaphragm. The diaphragm is a muscle that allows deep abdominal breathing, which moves the blood and lymph.

If the colon gets backed up and starts putrefying, fermenting and becoming gaseous the pressure will affect the rest of the body. Gas will push up on the diaphragm which restricts breathing and puts pressure on the heart giving pain.

In Chinese medicine the lungs and the colon are complementary; what happens to the colon affects the lungs.

Constipation and gas can cause back pain if the gas pushes up on the rib cage making the spine shift to one side or the other (throwing the back out of alignment) creating back pain.

The colon must stay unconstipated and free of gas to prevent backing up into the small intestine and other organs.

The lymphatic system must be kept clean at the microscopic capillary level in order to keep the blood stream purified. The microscopic level is where disease and aging begins.

We can't be healthy if our digestive system is a sick cesspool of constipating mucus and gas. V. E. Irons, an expert on colon health, points out that, "if there is CONSTIPATION then there is decay, fermentation and putrefication making the blood impure and thus poisoning the brain and nervous system creating depression and irritability. Impure blood will poison; the heart making you weak and listless, the lungs so the breath is foul, the digestive organs so we are distressed and bloated, the skin so it's dull and flaccid."

ENDO, MESO OR ECTOMORPH?

The body is naturally lean and flexible not fat, bloated and rigid like an obese person nor stout and dense like the football lineman. The wide receiver or swimmer is lean and agile just like the body is naturally eating a natural diet. A lean body with muscular definition is ideal or an ecto-meso hybrid and not the heavy, over-muscular body-builder look.

ARE YOU REALLY WELL NOURISHED?

Do you nourish yourself? Do you take the time and responsibility to make sure you get the right quality and quantity of food at the right time?

Nurture means to nurse or suckle, to promote the growth of, to support, maintain and feed. The word nature is very similar to the word nurture. A nurturer is one who helps the well-being and health of another.

Do you feed yourself well (especially men) now that you no longer are cared for by your mother? Do you really feed yourself well? Do you plan your meal times so you don't get low blood sugar mood swings and that feeling of weakness? The brain needs a lot of glucose.

Eat when hungry is the old Zen adage, but it really means eat when you start to feel weak. It's best to stop working or doing whatever you're doing when you start to feel weak and eat.

First we must know and accept that we are loved by God, then we can love ourselves completely and thereby love others as we love ourselves. Love yourself whole heartedly with warmth, caring and compassion because God the Father and Goddess the Mother loves you completely. If you don't love yourself you won't be able to treat others with love because it all flows out from you. Fall in love with your True Self, the Spirit Within.

HOW TO BINGE WITHOUT RUINING YOUR HEALTH

BINGES, CRAVINGS,
ADDICTIONS, RESTAURANTS

The transition diet is a very long process taking many years to offset the many years of wrong eating. At times one will get bored with the routine and want a change. Eating at a restaurant or ordering take-out is a good way to break the monotony during the early stages of the transition process. A Chinese or Thai dish that is based on stir-fried or steamed vegetables is a good choice and can be eaten with a large salad. Make sure to ask if the food is MSG free or else you can end up with a painful headache.

Many regular restaurants have vegetarian entrees and salad bars. Any vegetable based dish is good during the transition. This flexibility allows one to take a break from the routine and have something different in taste, texture and aroma.

It also allows one to socialize with friends and family during the long transition process. This will allow one not to feel so alien and strange around your family and friends, giving you the chance to gradually adapt them to your new way of eating. Sometimes you will get the urge to really binge out and have a ball. This is when going to a restaurant or ordering take-out can break the monotony.

As one's body gets more mucus free, the effect of the wrong foods will become quickly apparent as one gets a runny nose, blocked sinuses, earache, headache and starts to cough. You will see immediately the effect that binging has on your body and slowly you won't want to do it anymore. Painful, hard experience will gradually make you shy away from the wrong foods.

If you're addicted to ice cream or soy ice cream, a good transition recipe is to freeze peeled bananas and then blend them with berries and or carob powder to make a more natural ice cream.

If you are addicted to cake, cookies, candy and brownies try making carob "flour" (raw carob powder) goodies like brownies, fudge, cake and cookies. Combine raw carob powder with ripe bananas by mashing them together with a fork.

Using more powder will create a dryer mix and using less powder a more moist end product. It's better to make a moist, water rich product to prevent any constipating effects. You can even add a little purified or coconut water. Add natural vanilla powder for added flavoring. Shape the dough into a square and make it thick in order to make carob brownies.

A SAFER BINGE

If you feel you must binge on something try baked or grilled potatoes topped with grass-fed butter or a little avocado and seasoned with herb salt. Thin slice the potatoes and broil or bake them until golden brown.

Binging on three or more avocados will clog up the lymph and capillary tubes. Potatoes are alkaline and will pass through you easier and will leave little hangover pain the next day.

An all out avocado binge is very hard on the liver and really acidifies your system. Eat avocado with tomatoes, cucumbers and lemon juice to dilute the fat. Concentrated unsaturated fats as found in avocados and nuts rob your body of oxygen. Oxygen is needed by your cells to create bioelectric energy from glucose.

As Dr. C. Samuel West, D.N., N.D., author of The Golden Seven Plus One (1981), and a member of The International Society of Lymphology besides founder of the International Academy of Lymphology put it, "fats combine with oxygen and they form 'free radicals', which in turn, use up more available oxygen to form toxic peroxides that can damage and destroy cells. Peroxides will cause cells to mutate and mutated cells are highly cancerous. This helps explain how fats cause lack of oxygen and cancer."

Unsaturated "poly" and "mono" fats found in vegetable oils, even organic, cold pressed, extra virgin and refined olive oil, will form free radicals but saturated fats like grass-fed sour cream, butter and coconut oil, which are low in polyunsaturated fats, are stable.

Dr. West's findings about the importance of the lymphatic system in maintaining health is supported by the Textbook of Medical Physiology, Arthur C. Guyton M.D. (1996) author, the best selling physiology textbook in the world and quite possibly the most widely used medical textbook of any kind.

In 1981 Dr. West presented his findings before the International

Society of Lymphology which comprises top medical research scientists and heads of medical faculties worldwide.

Dr. West explains that the reason why you get sick eating just fruit is because it will pull excess sodium out, dissipate the clustered proteins and release toxins into the bloodstream too quickly. Eating potato soup will stop the elimination process and you feel good again.

His Lymphology course cited Ehret as "The Daddy of Transition".

A safer binge would be to use rye crisp bread (RYVITA and WASA are two well known brand names) with a little mashed avocado, jam or apple sauce spread on top. Dried organic mango, dates, raisins and prunes (better if soaked) are good treats for an occasional morning snack or they can be eaten with the salad.

If you really have strong cravings for old foods try chewing the food, tasting it well in your mouth, then spit it out without swallowing.

Some highly seasoned or chemical containing foods can be absorbed through the mucus membranes of the mouth, so be careful to avoid headaches. This method is better than swallowing the food and then vomiting it later. Eventually you will tire of this or become sick to your stomach just from having the food in your mouth. Be kind to yourself and give yourself enough time to slowly give up all these deeply ingrained, old food habits.

During the transition the craving for fat needs to be controlled and monitored. Natural dairy products like grass-fed butter, whole milk cheese and coconut oil have the healthiest forms of fat for our body, but that being said, they should be consumed moderately and combined with a higher proportion of vegetables.

Vegetable oils, with the exception of coconut oil, begin oxidizing and turning rancid the minute they are extracted. High quality olive oil comes in dark glass or cans to prevent rancidity. For the transition, raw sour cream, butter, coconut oil and a good quality olive oil are essential. Avocados are too high in polyunsaturated fats to be considered a healthy fat and also are too expensive or unavailable in some localities.

Saturated fats found in grass-fed dairy products are the best fats because they provide the fat soluble vitamins A, D, E and K and do not go rancid.

Raw Swiss cheese is the least mucus forming cheese and very high in calcium (224 mg in a one ounce portion and just 161 mg phosphorus). Fresh farmer's cheese (available at Mexican food markets) or cottage cheese are also good cheeses and less expensive. Cheese is a concentrated food and therefore needs to be diluted with a larger portion of vegetables and vegetable fruits (tomato, cucumber).

HELPFUL TRANSITION TIPS

Remember, if you are cleansing too fast, starchy vegetables (broccoli etc.) weather cooked or raw, will not solve the problem since they are not mucus forming. Cooked starches like potato and brown rice, which are mucus forming, need to be eaten.

Yam, sweet potato and squash are not mucus rich like potatoes are, rather they are mucus poor like carrots. Brussels sprouts and maize (corn) are acidic. Plantain (a big, green starchy banana that is eaten cooked) is not a good cooked starch.

Uncooked starchy vegetables (cauliflower, broccoli, cabbage, eggplant and zucchini) contain anti-nutrients such as alkylrescorcinols, alpha-amylase inhibitors and protease inhibitors damaging to human physiological systems. Small amounts of raw broccoli and cabbage are ok. Eating a lot of uncooked cabbage can inhibit the function of the thyroid gland.

Artichokes due to their starch content need to be cooked. Mint tea can be used to soothe the digestive tract. Chamomile is useful for calming the nerves.

Exercise is a necessary aid to the transition detoxification process. Weight training enlarges and shapes specific muscles. Running increases your cardio-vascular capacity and leg size. Bouncing on a mini-trampoline helps to detoxify the body faster by moving the lymphatic system.

Singing is excellent to loosen mucus in the lungs. Working in the garden is an excellent natural exercise. A multi-tiered, fruit tree, forest garden can provide all your food. Tall growing fruit trees form the highest level of the canopy with smaller growing fruit trees and berry shrubs forming the lower levels. Tomato, cucumber and bell pepper besides succulent vegetables like lettuce and spinach can be grown in the tree clearings.

HOW TO DO A ONE DAY
OR LONGER FAST

AN HERBAL LAXATIVE
MAKES IT A PLEASURE TO FAST

The key to fasting easily and pleasurably is to empty your bowels at the beginning of the fast. Without a toxic load in your intestine, your bloodstream is not re-contaminated by old waste, making it a pleasure to fast. If the intestines and digestive tract are free of old waste matter the body is then free to clean up its waste in other parts of the body. If the colon is constipated, the whole body will be constipated or backed up with old fecal matter. The colon is like the sewer of the house, if it's clogged up, the whole house will smell putrid.

Senna or cassia is a natural herb, not a harsh chemical, so it's gentler on your body. One can use bulk herbs by mixing a handful in 2 cups of water in a pan, then bring it to a boil, lower the flame and simmer until you have about one half cup of liquid. Filter out the leaf with a wire or plastic sieve. Use reverse osmosis filtered or distilled water if possible.

This will empty your intestines in about five hours making it much easier to fast. 2 or 3 cassia or senna teabags placed in a cup of hot water will also work, but not as well as the bulk herbs. Tablets of dried herbs don't work as well as a liquid solution of the herbs.

In an emergency, where the stool is solidified hard as a rock in the colon, a warm water enema could quickly dissolve the problem. But generally the herbal laxative is the preferred mode of emptying the bowels.

Enemas don't work as easily and as well as using senna. The herbal laxative purges the whole intestine system, whereas the enema usually only cleans out the lower part of the colon. Enemas are more complicated with the need for a special enema bag and tube.

To take an enema, hang the enema bag a few feet above you, lie down on your left side, insert the tube in the anus and allow the warm water to enter. Massage the water up the descending colon, then turn on your back, and then to the right side, making sure the water has entered in all parts of the colon. When one can no longer hold the water one lets the water go in the toilet.

Excessive use of the enema weakens the muscles of the colon making it hard to have a normal bowel movement without an enema.

Herbal laxatives don't create this weakening, allowing one to return to normal food stimulated bowel movements after the fast.

During a longer fast of 2 to 5 days or longer one can also take a laxative on the last day before breaking the fast to aid the elimination of old accumulated wastes. During a longer fast, toxic waste accumulates in the intestine, thus a laxative removes this waste without waiting for your first meal to stimulate a bowel movement.

WHEN TO FAST AND REDUCE
MUCUS FORMING FOODS

Gradually, after a few months on the transition, you can try a short one and a half day or 40 hour fast, taking only liquids like coconut water, vegetable juice and apple juice to see how toxic you are.

To do this fast, nearly 2 full days, just shy of 48 hours, first take the laxative senna, then skip breakfast, lunch and dinner and "break-fast" with solid food the next day at around 10 a.m. or 12 noon.

A fast will help clean you out better than a fruit fast, since the toxins are not stirred up on coconut water or juice like they are eating fresh fruit, which allows the body to eliminate better. Then, after the fast, one can begin reducing the amount of mucus forming foods and increasing raw salads and fruits.

After some time your diet will seem too heavy and one can gradually move toward a mucuslean diet (vegetables/fruit both raw and cooked and protein/fat but no or rarely cooked starches) by slowly removing the pasta, brown rice, potatoes and crisp bread.

First stop eating cooked starch at one of your meals each day, then when you're ready (it may take many months or even years) stop eating cooked starch altogether. After giving up starch you can slowly give up mayonnaise, poultry and fish to become a lacto-vegetarian.

SHORT FASTS CAN HELP
A HEALING CRISIS

During an elimination crisis such as a severe cold, fasting on or-

ange juice, pineapple juice, apple juice or lemonade made with purified or distilled water, a little lemon juice and a natural sweetener
(stevia, honey, maple syrup), can help speed up the elimination.

Slowing down an acute elimination crisis would be just prolonging
the symptoms causing greater stress and aging to the body. It's more
logical to fast on freshly extracted orange, pineapple or vegetable
juice, lemonade, bottled commercial juice and herb tea until the symptoms pass and then with this newly clean body start a new diet with
less mucus forming food.

Clean out the bowels with the herbal laxative senna first and then
let the body clean house. The common cold and the flu are really nature's blessing helping you take out the old garbage.

Germs and viruses live off of mucus and toxic waste products that
have accumulated in the body, but are not the cause of a cold or the
flu. The cause is the body's effort to rid itself of excess mucus and
toxic waste products.

FASTING, FALSE SEX AROUSAL, INDIGESTION

If you are really under weight and weak, a long fast or even any
fasting at all, would be weakening to your overall system. It's best to
fast when you are strong enough and clean enough to endure a
fast comfortably.

Another point to remember is that toxins and excess waste mate-
rials create an acid condition, which tends to irritate the sex glands
creating a false sexual arousal leading to sex obsession.

Whenever you detect the signs of toxicity (a sore throat, runny
nose, earaches, acne) just do a short fast or reduce mucus forming
foods to restore the balance. Remember to use the herb senna, also
called cassia, to empty the colon, making it easier to fast. Senna in
bulk herb form is the most effective.

Indigestion and gas can often be overcome by reducing the quantity eaten. Too much food strains the digestive enzymes so they can't
digest everything in the stomach, resulting in undigested food particles which cause pain, distension and gas.

That being said, remember to eat enough to have a bowel movement right after each meal. Reducing the number of food combinations, will also help alleviate indigestion problems.

ARE YOU TOXIC?

No offence, but do your pits smell like the pits? Does your pooh stink, your face break out, your tonsils ache, your ears feel plugged? These are signs that it's time to take out the garbage. You've overloaded your system and you need to wash your cellular clothes.

Even eating transition foods you can get toxic by overeating on mucus forming foods.

A moratorium on all eating is in order. Just drink vegetable juice or fruit juice or coconut water or watermelon juice (blended then filtered). Drinking enough liquid fills the stomach so you don't get hunger pangs, making it easier to fast.

When the cleansing reaction comes, fill up on vegetable juice, fruit juice or coconut water and go lie down to help the body process its poisons.

Dinner to dinner is 24 hours. Saturday you ate a big meal for dinner, so you fast or don't eat, just sip liquids all Sunday until dinnertime and then eat your regular meal, or if you feel good and strong fast until the next day, breaking the fast at noon. This longer 42 hour fast will do you more good because you are fasting overnight which allows the body to heal itself during sleep or the dormant period of absolute rest.

A long fast, lasting more than a day or two is useful only for those who have been in transition for a good period of time, because it speeds up the elimination rate considerably.

If you are still very toxic and you fast, you will overload your system causing irritability. A weekly fast of 36-42 hours is a very good habit to practice after you have been on the transition for a while.

Laxatives like senna or cassia tea will empty the bowels making the fast easier. Break the fast with vegetables if you are just beginning to fast, and fruits as you get more cleaned out. As one gets more purified, longer fasts of two or three days or longer can be experimented with.

MEAL PLANS

TRANSITION DIET MEAL PLAN
MONDAY

The Transition diet has plenty of cooked and raw vegetables, cooked starches, dairy and eggs to slow down the elimination process as opposed to the target high fruit and vegetable, lacto-vegetarian diet which is mostly fresh, living fruits, vegetables and cultured milk products. A semi-vegetarian diet adds moderate amounts of meat, fish, seafood and poultry to the lacto-vegetarian diet.

BREAKFAST:
Green Salad with Yogurt Dressing
String Bean, Squash and Eggplant Stew
Baked "French Fry" Potatoes

Green Salad: 2 grated carrots, red leaf lettuce leaves, 1/2 bunch spinach, 1 medium tomato, 1 cup raw homemade yogurt, 1 tablespoon spirulina
Stew: Kabocha squash 1/4 medium, 2 cups string beans, 1 medium eggplant, 2 medium tomatoes, 1 teaspoon Olive Oil, 1 medium white onion, clove garlic
Potato: 1 large potato sliced like French fries then baked or broiled 1/4 teaspoon salt
Note: If you don't have hard physical labor to do or you are not hungry eat the soup in the morning instead of for dinner.

LUNCH:
Green Salad (as above)
Grilled in Coconut Oil or Olive Oil: Broccoli, Onion, Bell Pepper, Cauliflower, Zucchini
Whole Wheat Lasagna
Lasagna: One portion

DINNER:
Hot Raw Vegetable Soup
2 cucumbers, 2 medium tomatoes, 3 large celery stalks, 2 medium carrots, 1/2 bunch spinach, 1 tablespoon spirulina, 3 cloves garlic grated in sieve. Heat until it's hot to your testing finger but not scalding. Sprinkle spirulina powder on top of the soup.

NUTRITIONAL ANALYSIS:
TRANSITION DIET MEAL PLAN
MONDAY

Percentage of calories derived from:

fat: 25%

protein: 20%

carbohydrates: 55%

Calorie Information

Total Calories 2442 %DV (Percent Daily Value)

Total Fat 70 g 108%DV

Total Omega-3 fatty acids 2158 mg

Total Omega-6 fatty acids 5714 mg

Protein 143 g 286%DV

Vitamin A 144,148 IU 2528%DV

Vitamin C 643 mg 1072%

Vitamin E (Alpha Tocopherol) 23.2 mg 116%

Vitamin K 3017 mcg 3771%

Thiamin 3.4 mg 228%

Riboflavin 4.5 mg 263%

Niacin 30.1 mg 151%

Vitamin B6 6.1 mg 307%

Folate 1835 mcg 459%

Vitamin B12 3.6 mcg 60%

Pantothenic Acid 12.2 mg 122%

Calcium 2093 mg 209%

Iron 40.8 mg 226%

Magnesium 984 mg 246%

Phosphorus 2632 mg 263%

Potassium 12822 mg 366%

Sodium 6186 mg 258%

Zinc 16.2 mg 108%

Copper 4.6 mg 232%

Manganese 10.4 mg 521%

Selenium 138 mcg 197%

Cholesterol 138 mg 46%

5459 total grams food of which 4845 grams is water or 88.8% water.

B-12 is only 60% of the Daily Value and can be supplemented using the methyl form.

Analysis: NutritionData from Self magazine

TRANSITION DIET MEAL PLAN
TUESDAY

BREAKFAST:
Pineapple slice
Papaya
Strawberries
Apple
Yogurt
Eaten sequentially one after another. Yogurt is eaten last
Or fast on liquids: coconut water, watermelon juice, vegetable juice

LUNCH:
Sauteed Cauliflower Soup
Green Salad With Mayonnaise Or Yogurt Dressing
Brown Rice

DINNER:
Green Salad With Italian Dressing
Vegetable Shish Kabob
Baked French Fries

TRANSITION DIET MEAL PLAN
WEDNESDAY

BREAKFAST:
Orange Juice 6-12 oz. or Coconut water,
Vegetable juice or Hot Raw Soup
If hungry or tired have:
Papaya
Strawberries
Apple
Yogurt

LUNCH:
Cauliflower Cream Soup
Green Salad With Mayonnaise Or Yogurt-Spirulina Dressing
Steamed Kabocha Squash
Baked Potato

DINNER:
Green Salad With Italian Dressing
Vegetable Shish Kabob
Baked French Fries

TRANSITION DIET MEAL PLAN
THURSDAY

BREAKFAST:
Cantalope

Eat the whole fruit or juice it in your mouth spitting out the pulp or use a juicer. You will detoxify quicker if you take only liquids in the morning (before 10:30 a.m.). If you need to do hard physical labor then eat plenty of whole fruit followed by yogurt and some cheese.

LUNCH:
Green Salad With Cultured Milk Dressing
Steamed Kabocha Squash
Rye Crisp Bread

DINNER:
Green Salad With Italian Dressing
Lasagna
Brown Rice

TRANSITION DIET MEAL PLAN
FRIDAY

BREAKFAST:
Watermelon juice 16 oz. (if you feel like only taking liquids)
Blend the watermelon flesh without seeds in a blender and then filter through a sieve.
or eat one after the other:
Watermelon
Papaya
Apple
Yogurt

LUNCH:
Green Salad With Yogurt and Spirulina Dressing
Steamed Artichokes
Brown Rice

DINNER:
Green Salad With Avocado Dressing
Steamed Broccoli
Whole Wheat Lasagna

Note: Check the recipes section for a detailed explanation of how to prepare these dishes.

TRANSITION DIET MEAL PLAN
SATURDAY

BREAKFAST:
Grated Apple With Cinnamon And Honey
On cold mornings warm it to body temperature (around 100 degrees
F) on the stove, stirring constantly to avoid burning.
Yogurt
Slice of cheese

LUNCH:
Green Salad
Grilled Vegetables
Mashed Potatoes

DINNER:
Lettuce Leaf Burritos
Cauliflower Cream Soup
Brown Rice
Green Pea Guacamole

TRANSITION DIET MEAL PLAN
SUNDAY

BREAKFAST:
Fresh Cantalope As Much As You Care To Eat
Followed by Yogurt

LUNCH:
Green Salad With Mayonnaise Or Yogurt and Avocado Dressing,
String Beans, Squash and Eggplant Stew
Brown Rice

DINNER:
Eat Out At A Vegetarian Restaurant

Or visit Sizzler, the famous steak place in the USA, which has a good
buffet salad bar. They have a good selection of salads, vegetable based
dishes and rice, pasta and potato.

Or do a 40 hour fast using senna leaf to clean out your digestive system (kind of like changing the oil in your car, do it every 3,000-6,000
miles and the engine will run smoother and last much longer).

THE LACTO-VEGETARIAN MEAL PLAN

The lacto-vegetarian diet consists of fresh, living fruits, vegetables and grass-fed, raw dairy products. Starchless vegetables include lettuce, celery, spinach, parsley, dandelion greens, kohlrabi, kale, cabbage, tomatoes, cucumbers and bell peppers. Carrots, beets and radishes can contain inorganic earth elements and are used just for the transition. It is better to use the more purified, earth element free, solar charged, above ground vegetables like celery, kohlrabi (delicious grated), lettuce and spinach.

Eat plenty of juicy fruits avoiding too many highly acidic fruits like pineapple and citrus and overly sweet fruit like watermelon, dates and bananas.

Eat plenty of grass-fed, raw cultured milk products (cottage cheese, cheese, butter, yogurt, sour cream).

This diet is healthier than a vegetarian diet based on cooked grains, cooked beans, cooked and raw vegetables, sprouts, fruit, milk products and eggs, seeds and nuts because it is not mucus forming and has a very low polyunsaturated and monounsaturated fat content.

Steamed or cooked vegetables are best mixed with at least 50% raw vegetables to get the raw food enzymes working to digest your food.

Have a drink first if thirsty like young coconut water, vegetable juice or watermelon juice then eat fruit sequentially one after another starting with the juiciest fruit first, then wait about 15 minutes and have vegetables and cultured dairy products.

LACTO-VEGETARIAN MEAL PLAN
MONDAY

BREAKFAST:
Eat sequentially one after the other:
Slice of Pineapple (thick, 84 gms)
One Hawaiian Papaya
10 medium size Strawberries
1 medium Apple sliced
Two cups yogurt

LUNCH:
One medium Apple
10 medium size Strawberries
One Hawaiian Papaya
One banana then wait 15 minutes before having:
Salad with Yogurt Dressing:
Red Leaf Lettuce, Grated Carrot,
Sliced Tomato, 1 cup Yogurt

DINNER:
Lettuce Leaf Sandwiches:
Fill a lettuce leaf with
Farmer's Cheese,
Sliced Tomato, Sliced Onion

NUTRITIONAL ANALYSIS:
LACTO-VEGETARIAN MEAL PLAN
MONDAY

Percentage of calories derived from:
fat: 30%
protein: 19%
carbohydrates: 51%

Calorie Information
Total Calories 1700
Fats %DV   (%DV Percent Daily Value)
Total Fat 59 g   91% DV
Total Omega-3 fatty acids 839 mg
Total Omega-6 fatty acids 1981 mg

Protein 80.5 g 161%DV

Vitamin A 49,239 IU 985%DV
Vitamin C 480 mg 800%
Vitamin E (Alpha Tocopherol) 7.7 mg 38%
Vitamin K 504 mcg 630%
Thiamin 1.1 mg 71%
Riboflavin 2.1 mg 123%
Niacin 9.0 mg 45%
Vitamin B6 2.4 mg 120%
Folate 552 mcg 138%
Vitamin B12 3.8 mcg 63%
Pantothenic Acid 6.6 mg 66%

Calcium 1809 mg 181%
Iron 19.1 mg 50%
Magnesium 346 mg 87%
Phosphorus 1708 mg 171%
Potassium 5347 mg 153%
Sodium 1864 mg 78%
Zinc 10.2 mg 68%
Copper 1.1 mg 56%
Manganese 3.8 mg 189%
Selenium 57.4 mcg 82%
Water 2213 grams or 88% of the total 2512 gram weight

Analysis: NutritionData from Self magazine

A natural, food-grown multi-vitamin supplement would fill any deficit in vitamins and minerals.

LACTO-VEGETARIAN MEAL PLAN
TUESDAY

BREAKFAST:
Fruits of your choice eaten sequentially, wait 15 minutes then eat:
Lettuce Leaf Sandwiches:
Romaine or Head Lettuce Leaves
Natural Cheese Slices, Yogurt,
Sliced Tomato, Spinach,
Sliced Onion

LUNCH:

Plums, Peaches, Cherries
eaten Sequentially, then wait around 15-20 minutes and eat:
Pizza Salad with Yogurt, Slice of Cheese

Sequential eating means eating one variety of fruit resting and then eating another variety of fruit. This way the stomach is not confused as to how to digest different varieties of fruit. Even watermelons and other melons can be eaten sequentially if you eat them first and then wait a while before eating a different variety of fruit. About 20 minutes after eating a lot of fruit, you can feel weak, that is when to have your vegetable salad and cultured milk. Having fruit then vegetables with protein in the morning and for lunch gives you more energy and strength to work hard during the day. Dinner can be a light meal of fruit and if needed some yogurt after but not mixed with the fruit or if you are thirsty just drink coconut water, apple juice, vegetable juice or have hot raw soup.

DINNER:
Raw Apple Sauce
Yogurt
Coarse grate organic apple and add powdered or grated cinnamon, honey and raisin. Can be stored in glass bottles.

LACTO-VEGETARIAN MEAL PLAN
WEDNESDAY

BREAKFAST:
Slice of Watermelon
A few Strawberries
One half Hawaiian Papaya
One banana
Eaten sequentially
followed 15-20 minutes later by:
Green Salad With Spirulina-Yogurt Dressing
With Spinach, Lettuce
Grated cabbage, Celery,
Tomato

LUNCH:
Fruit of your choice, then wait about 15-20 minutes and have:
Cabbage Leaf Sandwiches:
Cabbage Leaves
Natural Cheese, Yogurt,
Sliced Tomato, Spinach,
Sliced Onion

DINNER:
Coconut water, fresh vegetable juice or wheat grass juice.
Or have Fruit In Season. Follow with yogurt if needed.

LACTO-VEGETARIAN MEAL PLAN
THURSDAY

BREAKFAST:
Coconut water or vegetable juice
Strawberries
Papaya
Apple
Eaten sequentially
Greek Salad: Cucumbers, Tomatoes, Bell Peppers,
Black Olives, Oregano, Lemon Juice, Feta Cheese

LUNCH:
Watermelon
Eat The Amount Your Body Tells You To Eat
Lettuce Salad with Yogurt Dressing

Whether you eat more vegetables or more fruit depends on your body
and the season. In summer you will want to eat more fruit, so you
have to make sure you get enough calcium, magnesium and vitamin
D to build strong teeth and bones.

DINNER:
Watermelon Juice
Fruit in season, followed by yogurt if needed.

LACTO-VEGETARIAN MEAL PLAN
FRIDAY

BREAKFAST:
Coconut water or vegetable juice
Mango
Grated Apple With Cinnamon

Eaten sequentially, one after the other
Eat just one mango because it's a sweet fruit
Wait about 10-15 minutes, enough for the fruit to digest, and then have vegetables;
Pizza Salad, Bieler's Soup
If you want a complete living foods diet, skip the cooked soup.

LUNCH:
Celery, Carrot, Spinach Juice
Fresh Figs 2-4 lbs.
Lettuce Sandwich: Romaine or Head Lettuce Leaves, Tomato Slice, White Onion Slice, Red Bell Pepper Slice, Cheese

During the summer there are usually a few big fig trees around that are overloaded with figs and nobody is picking them, or if you see a tree loaded with fruit just ask the owners and they usually let you pick to your heart's content.

DINNER:
Coconut Water
Some Hawaiian Papaya, a few Strawberries, 1/2 an Apple
Salad: Lettuce, Grated Cabbage, Tomatoes,
Bell Peppers, Black Olives, Raw Yogurt
Sprinkle a teaspoon or two of Spirulina on top of the yogurt

LACTO-VEGETARIAN MEAL PLAN
SATURDAY

BREAKFAST:
Orange Juice 12 Oz. (a cup and a half)
Hot Raw Vegetable Soup

LUNCH:
Mangoes
Apples

On Saturday many people leave the house on excursions, so bring enough fruit for the whole day. While away from the house eat mono fruit meals (only one type of fruit) whenever tired and hungry and save the vegetables for dinner

DINNER:
Vegetable juice: wheat grass,
dandelion greens,
celery, cucumber
Pizza Salad with
Yogurt and Spirulina dressing

LACTO-VEGETARIAN MEAL PLAN
SUNDAY

BREAKFAST:
Mango
Apple Slices
Eaten sequentially, one after the other
Eat just one mango because it's a sweet fruit
Wait about 15 minutes then follow with a Pizza Salad

LUNCH:
Coconut Water
Fresh Figs 2-4 lbs.
Plums

If you are out and about on Sunday just eat fruit and wait till dinner to eat vegetables

During the summer there are usually a few big fruit trees around in people's yards or in abandoned orchards that are overloaded with fruit and free for the asking.

DINNER:
Salad: Lettuce, Grated Cabbage, Tomatoes, Bell Peppers, Black Olives, Dressed with Raw Yogurt

If you ever feel bloated, constipated or have gas, do a one day fast with the herbal laxative senna. Skip breakfast, lunch, dinner and break the fast the next day. The whole day feast on coconut water, fruit juices like apple or pineapple, fresh vegetable juices and hot, raw vegetable soup.

THE SEMI-VEGETARIAN
OR FLEXITARIAN MEAL PLAN

A semi-vegetarian diet, also called a flexitarian diet is healthier if based on fruits, vegetables and cultured milk and not rice, bread. pasta and beans. Select meat, poultry and fish that are the most toxin-free. Lamb meat is usually grass-fed and some beef is grass-fed if looked for in natural food stores. Chicken, even organic, is usually grain-fed, so look for free range chicken. Grain-fed chicken and beef makes their fat content high in the highly unstable polyunsaturated fats. Eat low fat (low in the free-radical forming polyunsaturated fats) and low mercury seafood like scallops, shrimp, snow crab, sole, tilapia, flounder, white fish, whiting and cod. Chum and pink salmon are low fat and low mercury if wild Alaskan or Pacific. Atlantic, coho, king and sockeye are higher fat salmon.

SEMI-VEGETARIAN MEAL PLAN
MONDAY

BREAKFAST:
Eat sequentially one after the other:
Papaya
Strawberries
Apple
Yogurt

LUNCH:
Sauteed Cauliflower Soup
Green Salad With Clabbered Milk Dressing
Brown Rice
Piece of Free Range Organic Baked Chicken

DINNER:
Green Salad With Cottage Cheese Dressing
Baked French Fries
Baked or Grilled Alaskan Chum Salmon

NUTRITIONAL ANALYSIS:
SEMI-VEGETARIAN DIET MEAL PLAN
MONDAY

Percentage of calories derived from fat: 31%
Percentage of calories derived from protein: 22%
Percentage of calories derived from carbohydrates: 47%

Calorie Information
Total Calories 2140
Fats %DV   (%DV Percent Daily Value)
Total Fat 76.4 g   117% DV
Total Omega-3 fatty acids   1426 mg
Total Omega-6 fatty acids   3625 mg

Protein 121 g   243% DV

Vitamin A 66253 IU 1325% DV
Vitamin C 407 mg 678%
Vitamin E (Alpha Tocopherol) 8.0 mg 40%
Vitamin K 530 mcg 662%
Thiamin 1.7 mg 111%
Riboflavin 2.9 mg 168%
Niacin 26.7 mg 133%
Vitamin B6 3.4 mg 171%
Folate 701 mcg 175%
Vitamin B12 12.5 mcg 208%
Pantothenic Acid 10.2 mg 102%

Calcium 1546 mg 155%
Iron 14.9 mg 83%
Magnesium 436 mg 109%
Phosphorus 2138 mg 214%
Potassium 7152 mg 204%
Sodium 2725 mg 114%
Zinc 10.9 mg 72%
Copper 1.6 mg 78%
Manganese 3.8 mg 188%
Selenium 115 mcg 165%
Water 2971 grams or 86% of the total 3458 gram weight

Analysis: NutritionData from Self magazine
A high quality food based or food grown multi-vitamin supplement would
fill any deficit in vitamins and minerals.

SEMI-VEGETARIAN MEAL PLAN
TUESDAY (MEAT-FREE)

BREAKFAST:
Eat sequentially one after the other:
Orange Juice 6-12 oz. or Coconut water
Papaya
Strawberries
Apple
Yogurt

LUNCH:
Cauliflower Cream Soup
Green Salad With Mayonnaise Or Yogurt-Spirulina Dressing
Steamed Kabocha Squash
Baked Potato

DINNER:
Green Salad With Italian Dressing
Vegetable Shish Kabob
Baked French Fries

SEMI-VEGETARIAN MEAL PLAN
WEDNESDAY

BREAKFAST:
Eat sequentially one after the other:
One Hawaiian Papaya
10 medium size Strawberries
1 medium Apple sliced
Two cups yogurt

LUNCH:
One medium Apple
10 medium size Strawberries
One Hawaiian Papaya
One banana then wait 15 minutes before having:
Salad with Cottage Cheese Dressing:
Red Leaf Lettuce, Grated Carrot,
Sliced Tomato, 1 cup Cottage Cheese
Roast, Free Range Organic Chicken

DINNER:
Lettuce Leaf Sandwiches:
Fill a lettuce leaf with
Cheese, Sliced Tomato, Sliced Onion
A Serving of Grilled or Baked Chum or Pink Salmon
(Pacific or Alaskan)

SEMI-VEGETARIAN MEAL PLAN
THURSDAY

BREAKFAST:
Coconut water
Strawberries
Apples
Mango
Eaten sequentially, one after the other
Eat mango last and just one because it's a sweet fruit
Wait about 15 minutes then follow with a Grated Carrot and Lettuce
Salad with Yogurt Dressing, Bieler's Soup

LUNCH:
Coconut Water
Fresh Figs 2-4 lbs.
During the summer there are usually a few big fig trees around that
are overloaded with figs and free for the asking.
Free Range Organic Chicken or Turkey Toasted Bread Sandwiches

DINNER:
Salad: Lettuce, Grated Cabbage, Grated Carrot, Tomatoes, Bell Peppers, Black Olives, Dressed with Raw Yogurt
Lamb Chops

SEMI-VEGETARIAN MEAL PLAN
FRIDAY (MEAT-FREE)

BREAKFAST:
Grated Apple With Cinnamon And Honey
On cold mornings warm it to body temperature (around 100 degrees
F) on the stove, stirring constantly to avoid burning
Yogurt
Slice of cheese

LUNCH:
Green Salad
Grilled Vegetables
Mashed Potatoes

DINNER:
Cabbage Leaf Burritos
Cauliflower Cream Soup
Brown Rice
Green Pea Guacamole

SEMI-VEGETARIAN MEAL PLAN
SATURDAY

BREAKFAST:
Pineapple slice
Papaya
Strawberries
Apple
Yogurt

LUNCH:
Sauteed Cauliflower Soup
Green Salad With Clabbered Milk Dressing
Brown Rice
Piece of Free Range Organic Roasted Chicken

DINNER:
Green Salad With Italian Dressing
Vegetable Shish Kabob
Baked French Fries
Baked or Pan Fried Tilapia or Sole (avoid frying fish in vegetable oil
due to the excess polyunsaturated fat, instead use coconut oil)

SEMI-VEGETARIAN MEAL PLAN
SUNDAY (MEAT-FREE)

BREAKFAST:
Fresh Cantalope As Much As You Care To Eat
Followed by Yogurt

LUNCH:
Green Salad With Yogurt Dressing
String Beans, Squash and Eggplant Stew
Brown Rice

DINNER:
Eat Out At A Vegetarian Restaurant
Or visit Sizzler restaurant or other similar place that has a good buffet
salad bar and just eat meatless vegetarian dishes

RECIPES

DRINKS
For the transition, lacto-vegetarian
and semi-vegetarian diets

Young Coconut Water: Take a young, green/brown coconut and puncture the top with a knife. Stick in a straw and enjoy. Sweeten coconut water with lemon juice, honey or stevia and make lemonade. White sugar, brown sugar and cane juice sugar can rot your teeth. Processed, extracted sugar is like dried fruit, it rots the teeth due to the super concentrated sugars which drain minerals out of the teeth and bones and due to missing enzymes. Raw sugar cane/juice is ok on the teeth.

Vegetable Juice: Freshly extracted vegetable juice is mineralizing. See the chapter on vegetable juices for detailed information. Bottled vegetable juice can also be used. Filter the pulp to ease digestion.

Watermelon Juice: Scoop out the watermelon flesh without seeds then blend. Strain out the pulp.

Herb Tea: Use coconut water then add the herb teabag flavor of your choice; mint, chamomile etc., sweeten with raw honey or stevia.

Whey: When you make cottage cheese you will have extra, non-acidic whey. Avoid acidic, high lactic acid whey liquid that tastes acidic.

Papaya Milkshake: Remove the seeds from a papaya and scoop out the flesh into a blender or bowl. Add 3 ripe bananas (enough to thicken) and blend until it turns creamy. Add berries for a berry shake or carob powder for a "chocolate" shake. The above drinks are instantly absorbed but this smoothie takes time to digest.

Banana Ice Cream Milkshakes: Bananas can be peeled and frozen in the freezer. Put a plate under them so the banana doesn't stick to the freezer. Put one large frozen banana in a smoothie mixed with other unfrozen bananas and papaya, diluting the frozen banana. Frozen bananas eaten alone can cause indigestion.

Orange juice: Juice only ripe, sweet oranges using an electric citrus juicer or by hand, add 50% mandarin for a different flavor. Filter one time with a sieve to remove some of the pulp which can interfere with the rapid "15 minute blood transfusion" digestion.

Pineapple juice: Choose ripe, good smelling, deeply colored fruit and avoid acidic, green and fragrance-free fruit. Use a good, high quality juicer like the Omega chrome finish juicer. Cut off the scales and ends with a serrated knife, then slice lengthwise. Use a sieve once to filter. out the pulp. Store in the refrigerator and sip when thirsty.

VEGETABLE DRESSINGS
For the transition, lacto-vegetarian
and semi-vegetarian diets

Yogurt Dressing: Use raw homemade yogurt that has been skimmed of fat. Use about one cup of yogurt per individual salad and place on top of the prepared salad vegetables. Add one or two tablespoons of yogurt cream that you skimmed for extra creaminess. If desired add some grated cheese on top. Mix the salad well so all the salad vegetables are coated.

Italian Tomato Sauce: Sauté a large chopped onion and a diced piece of garlic in natural coconut oil until the onion turns clear. Add a heaping teaspoon of tomato paste, a large diced tomato and bell pepper and simmer. For large batches just increase the quantities of each ingredient.

Basic Oil, Lemon Juice and Salt Dressing: Wash the lettuce well then add a few teaspoons of lemon juice or seasoned rice vinegar or apple cider vinegar to the lettuce. Then add just a pinch of natural salt and toss. Add just enough olive oil, usually one or two teaspoons, to give it flavor without adding too much fat. Use garlic if salt sensitive.

Avocado Dressing: Blend in a blender or mash in a bowl with a fork, one quarter avocado with a little seasoned rice vinegar or apple cider vinegar or lemon juice, soy sauce, purified water (just enough, not too watery) and a bit of onion and garlic.

Onion, Lemon Juice and Oil Dressing: Cut a white onion in thin, round slices with a sharp knife. Cover the onion in a natural salt and let it stand for 15 minutes. This will remove the hot, burning qualities of the onion. Wash the chopped onion in cold water to remove most of the salt then moisten with olive oil and season with a little lemon juice. Add the prepared onion to lettuce and toss.

Italian, Vinegar, Honey and Olive Oil Dressing: Take equal parts balsamic or red wine vinegar and honey. Add just enough olive oil to give it flavor. Add two garlic pieces smashed with a knife.

VEGETABLE RECIPES
Salad and Sandwich Recipes
for the Lacto-Vegetarian Diet
The Cooked Food Recipes Are
for the Transition,
Semi-Vegetarian Diet and
Moderate Lacto-Vegetarian Diet

Pizza Salad:

Ingredients:

Lettuce	1/4 head of Romaine, green leaf, head
Spinach	One handful
Tomato	2 medium
Greek olives	2 or more
Red onion	One small
Garlic	One large clove or 2 medium cloves
Raw yogurt	One cup
Cheese,	4 ounces
Fresh Basil	A few leaves

Cheese and yogurt give this salad a rich, creamy taste. Greens, like the many varieties of lettuce (bibb, head, red leaf, green leaf, oak leaf, romaine), spinach and celery and can be mixed together, well chopped.

Add chopped tomatoes, mashed Kalamata Greek olives, a little grated garlic and a squeeze of lemon. For variety sauté onions, garlic and tomato in coconut oil and add it on top of the salad.

The greens are all one group of foods, the tomatoes are another and the yogurt another. This makes three groups of food which combine and digest well together. The onions, olives, garlic and lemon juice are for flavor. For the dressing use raw homemade yogurt and grated cheese.

Pour on the skimmed homemade yogurt. Skimmed yogurt is when you skim off the fat of your homemade yogurt in order to have a reduced fat yogurt, which is lower in calories. Use the cream a little at a time. Heat the vegetables in a metal bowl on top of the range by stirring slowly until warm to hot but not cooked or steaming. Remove from the heat and grate some cheese on top so it melts on top.

Carrot And Cabbage Cole Slaw Salad:

Ingredients:

Carrots	1 large finely grated
Cabbage	1 small cut piece, roughly grated
Lettuce	1 or 2 leaves of Romaine
Spinach	One handful
Tomato	1/2 chopped finely

Optional: Beet 1/2 cup finely or roughly grated

Dressing:
Yogurt   1 cup per person
Yogurt Cream 1 or 2 tablespoons

Optional:
Olive Oil   1 teaspoon
Avocado   1/8 to 1/4 for extra creaminess

    Take the grated carrot and cabbage and mix together in a salad bowl. Add the optional ingredients, if desired and mix. Add the yogurt and yogurt cream and mix thoroughly. If desired add the optional olive oil and avocado for extra creaminess. Eat with a good slice of cheese on the side or grated on top.

Pizza (transition recipe): A fast pizza can be made using toasted bread.
Ingredients:

Natural Cheese	1 medium slice
Yeast Bread	1 slice
Tomato	1 medium
Butter or Olive oil	1 tablespoon

    Lightly sauté the cheese slice and tomato slices and toast the bread. Place the melted cheese and tomato on the toast or just eat it without bread. Add torn basil leaves on top. For a sauce type pizza use the recipe, Italian Tomato Sauce and coat the bread first then add the melted cheese and topping like bell peppers, onions, sliced olives and basil. To make a traditional pizza buy a ready-made pizza crust or make the dough from scratch using flour. Here's a recipe:

Pizza Dough (transition recipe):
Ingredients: 3 1/2 to 4 cups bread flour, plus more for rolling (Note: Using bread flour will give you a much crisper crust. If you can't find bread flour, you can substitute it with all-purpose flour which will give you a chewier crust.)
1 teaspoon sugar
1 envelope instant dry yeast
2 teaspoons salt
1 1/2 cups water, 110 degrees F
2 tablespoons olive oil, plus 2 teaspoons

    Combine the bread flour, sugar, yeast and salt in a mixing bowl. Add the water and 2 tablespoons of the oil and beat by hand or in a mixer until the dough forms into a ball. If the dough is sticky, add additional flour, 1 tablespoon at a time, until the dough comes together in a solid ball. If the dough is too dry, add additional water, 1 tablespoon at a time.

Scrape the dough onto a lightly floured surface and gently knead into a smooth, firm ball. Grease a large bowl with the remaining 2 teaspoons olive oil, add the dough, cover the bowl with plastic wrap and put it in a warm area to let it double in size, about 1 hour.

Turn the dough out onto a lightly floured surface and divide it into 2 equal pieces. Cover each with a clean kitchen towel or plastic wrap and let them rest for 10 minutes. Yields 2 (14-inch) pizza crusts.

To cook on a grill; Heat your grill to medium-high. Using your hands, spread the pizza dough to form a 1/4-inch thick pizza. Brush one side with olive oil and put it, oil side down, onto the grill. Brush some more oil on the top and close the cover, if you have one. Cook until the bottom is browned and the top is set, about 5 minutes. Flip the crust over and cook on the other side until browned, about another 3 minutes. Remove from the heat and set aside until your guests arrive.

When your guests arrive or spread some tomato sauce onto the crust and top with grated mozzarella and your favorite toppings. Put the pizza back on the hot grill, close the cover if you have one, and cook until the cheese is melted and bubbling, about 5 to 6 minutes.

Hamburger: There's nothing like a hamburger with its lettuce, tomato and onion taste sensations.
Ingredients:

Romaine or Head Lettuce	4-6 large leaves
Ripe Red Tomatoes	2 large
White Onion	1 large
Cheese, Cottage or Raw	1/2 cup
Avocado	A few slices

Layer the lettuce slice with cheese, sliced tomatoes, avocado and white onion. Also can be made with toasted yeast-raised bread.

Eggplant Pizza:
Ingredients:

Eggplant, dark black	1 large or extra large
Tomato	1 large
Cottage/Raw Cheese	half cup
White Onion	1 large
Olive oil	refined/virgin type
Oregano dried	teaspoon

Slice a large, dark, black colored (this means it's ripe) eggplant lengthwise into half inch thick slices, then steam or slow cook until slightly soft. Avoid cooking the eggplant in water to prevent it from getting soggy. Then grill at low heat briefly to make it crisp. Spread some homemade Italian tomato sauce on top of the eggplant. Then place a layer of raw cottage cheese or raw cheese on top. Layer on top sliced fresh tomato, fresh bell peppers and onions. Season with dried oregano.

Steamed Potatoes:
Ingredients:
Potatoes   Yellow Finn, Russet or Red
    Steamed potatoes are a quick and easy food to prepare. Take a few small yellow potatoes or one or two big Russet or red potatoes and poke with a fork on all sides to speed cooking. Place in a covered steamer and cook until a fork, when stuck into the potato, will not hold the potato up, it slides right off. Avoid overcooking the potatoes which will result in a mushy consistency. Slice open the potato, if very large, to speed cooking time. Yogurt cream can be used to make potato salad by mixing with cubed steamed potatoes.

Mashed Potatoes:
Ingredients:
Potatoes   Yellow Finn, Russet or Red
    Steam the potatoes as described above and then mash them with a fork until they become creamy. Add yogurt cream if a more creamy consistency is desired. The mashed potato batter can also be shaped into a flat patty and grilled on a hot griddle, greased with coconut oil or butter, until browned on both sides to make potato pancakes.

Baked French Fries: Better tasting and healthier than oil-fried fries.
Ingredients:
Potatoes   3-4 medium
Butter or Coconut Oil One tablespoon
    Slice a potato lengthwise to make it French fry shaped. Then place on an oiled metal sheet and bake at 400 degrees F. until lightly browned on the outside. Season with butter and herb salt.

String Bean "French Fries":
Ingredients:
Tender String Beans   One pound
    Take fresh string beans, cut off the stems and steam, boil or slow cook (preserves all the nutrients) until tender. Their long shape and

taste gives you the feeling of eating French fries.

Whole Wheat Lasagna:
Ingredients:
Whole Wheat Lasagna Pasta
Tomato Sauce or Ripe Tomatoes
Cheese
Olive oil

Take whole wheat or whole wheat/spinach lasagna pasta and boil it until a dente or just when it gets soft, usually 15 minutes or so. Then take a metal or glass baking dish and lay down some cooked lasagna noodles on the bottom. Cover the pasta with tomato sauce (canned or homemade) and then cover this with grated mozzarella, ricotta, jack or Swiss cheese or raw, homemade cottage cheese. Keep layering until you reach the top and then bake at 375 F. until the cheese melts and the pasta becomes firm, which is usually about 20 minutes or so. Watch it so it doesn't overcook.

Green Pea Guacamole:
Ingredients:
Tender Green Peas   One pound or one half kilo

Boil one pound of fresh green peas in purified water using a covered pot until soft but not mushy. Filter out the hot, purified cooking water and set it aside. Blend the hot peas at low speed, slowly adding just enough hot cooking water to make it blend smoothly but still keeping it thick. Tastes delicious with no seasoning added. If desired blend in 2-3 garlic cloves, a little onion and lemon juice.

Cauliflower Cream Soup:
Ingredients:
Cauliflower   One large

Choose cauliflower that has tight, snowy white flowers. Avoid loose flowered and black spotted cauliflower. Cut whole cauliflower into quarters or individual flowers. Boil the cauliflower until slightly mushy (about 40 minutes), then blend with a little of the hot cooking water, a slice of onion, cilantro and a pinch of salt.

Sautéed Cauliflower Soup: A delicious transitional dish with egg
Ingredients:
Cauliflower	One large
Eggs	One egg
Whole Wheat flour	One tablespoon
Coconut Oil	Two tablespoons

Dried Achiote   One half teaspoon
Vegetarian soup cube One

Peel off the outer husk of the individual cauliflower stems, then cook in enough purified water to make them float. When soft roll them in egg beaten with a little wheat flour then sauté in two tablespoons oil until lightly browned. Add the sautéed cauliflower to the hot cook water and add a half teaspoon salt, a dash of achiote and a vegetarian soup cube. Delicious with carrot and cabbage coleslaw.

Tomato Soup:
Ingredients:

Tomatoes	4 medium
Olive Oil	2 tablespoons
Vegetarian Cube	1 cube, no msg
Purified Water	one half cup

Cut 4 tomatoes (per person) in quarters and put in the blender. Add a half cup reverse osmosis purified or distilled water, a vegetarian soup cube, 2 tablespoons olive oil and a little; powdered achiote, comino, garlic powder, salt. Liquefy. Filter the liquid, separate out the seeds, then cook 15 minutes on low heat. If watery add 1/2 teaspoon wheat flour dissolved in 1/2 cup cold water.

Hot Raw Vegetable Soup:
Ingredients:

Celery	3 stalks
Spinach	One half bunch
Tomatoes	2 medium
Carrots	3-4 medium
Red Bell Pepper	One medium
Cilantro	Handful
Cucumber	One half

Juice all the vegetables to make a quart of liquid. Filter three times through a fine sieve, the third time put 3 cloves of grated garlic in the sieve. Heat the liquid in a pan until hot, but not boiling. If you can stick your finger in it or sip it without it burning you the enzymes are still intact and it's still a raw, enzyme-rich food. Top with spirulina.

Dr. Bieler's Soup (author of; *Food Is Your Best Medicine*):
Ingredients:
1 pound String Beans
(potassium rich for the pancreas and salivary glands)
2 pounds Zucchini
(sodium rich for the liver)

One handful Parsley
Optional: 3 stalks celery
4-6 cups Purified (Reverse Osmosis or Distilled) Water
no salt is added

Bring the 4-6 cups water to a rapid boil. Cut up the string beans and zucchini into medium sized pieces. Add them to the boiling water and cook 6 minutes. Turn off the heat and then add a handful of chopped parsley. Scoop out the vegetables and place in a blender. Add some of the cooking water, the amount depends on how thick you want the soup, and blend until smooth. Serve hot. You could also steam the string beans and zucchini to preserve more of the nutrients. This soup was the main part of the diet that eradicated arthritis.

Grilled Vegetables:
Ingredients:

Eggplant	One small
Asparagus	4 stalks
Zucchini	3 medium
Red Bell Pepper	1 medium
Tomato	2 medium
Coconut Oil	1 Tablespoon

You will need a gas, electric or charcoal grill. Cut widthwise; eggplant, onion, zucchini, asparagus, tomato and red bell pepper into slices that will cook easily on the grill; not too thin or thick. Use coconut oil to grease the metal grill. Lightly season with herb salt. Add fresh, chopped basil if desired, for a different taste sensation. Grill the vegetables on low heat to avoid charring. This is a cooked food recipe for use in the transition and semi-vegetarian diets.

String Bean, Squash and Eggplant Stew:
Ingredients:

Tender green beans	One pound
Kabocha squash	One quarter squash
Eggplant	One medium
Tomato	3 medium
Onion, white	One medium

Look for high quality, dark green, tender green beans for the best flavor. Cut off the stems on both ends by laying them in a row with the ends lined up. Cut in half or quarters as desired or leave long. Add cubed squash, eggplant, diced tomato and diced onion sautéed in coconut oil to the pot. Use ripe, deep colored kabocha squash for the best taste possible. Boil in water or steam until tender and easy to bite into; a half hour or longer. Add a little olive oil and herb salt before cooking.

Broccoli and Asparagus:
Ingredients:

Broccoli	One head
Asparagus	One bunch

Use organically grown broccoli for the best flavor. Cut the whole broccoli head in quarters or in florets and steam or boil (with just a little water at the bottom) until tender. Cooking time depends on how you like your broccoli; slightly crisp or soft, so watch it carefully to cook it just right. Steam or boil the asparagus spears only long enough to make them slightly tender. Asparagus is high in folate.

FRUIT RECIPES
For the transition, lacto-vegetarian
and semi-vegetarian diets

Carob Fudge Brownies:
Ingredients:
Raw carob powder   One or two cups
Papaya   One Hawaiian or Small Mexican
Organic ripe bananas   Three or four
Raw honey   One teaspoon
Real vanilla powder   A dash

Mix with a fork raw carob powder with already blended papaya and banana. Bananas make it creamy and papaya gives it moisture. Add carob powder until the mixture is just right, not too moist and not too dry. Add natural vanilla powder to enhance the flavor. For the best flavor use real, low heat processed, raw carob powder and not the toasted kind. Shape the batter into a rounded loaf to make carob bread. Mix the dry carob powder with enough papaya or banana in order to make a moist batter. If it's too dry, it'll cause constipation.

Raw Grated Apple And Cinnamon:
Ingredients:
Grated Apple 2-3 apples per person

Mix in a dash of ground cinnamon and raw grated ginger. Add mashed, ripe banana if desired. Warm on the stove if it's a cold day.

Hot Apple Pie:
Ingredients:
Apples   2 medium
Cinnamon   Dash
Honey   One teaspoon

Take an organic, ripe apple and slice it in half inch slices. Place the apple on the cutting board on its side and slice it in many thin rounds. On top of each slice sprinkle a little cinnamon and honey. Steam the apple rounds until soft but not soggy or too soft. Let the steam soften the apple. Take out the slices and place them on a plate and eat them slice by slice or mash the pieces together into a fruit compote. Add extra cinnamon and honey on top if needed.

FRUIT COMBINING

Sweet fruits can be eaten as mono-meals (for example only apples) or they can be eaten sequentially; eating one fruit at a time before eating another variety. For instance you could start the morning with blackberries, then wait a few minutes and eat some plums, then a guava, then some figs, then a half a papaya and finish with grated apple topped with cinnamon. Only after eating watermelon or other melons, being mostly water, do you have to wait a few minutes before eating another fruit. 15 minutes later you can eat a vegetable salad.

Non-sweet fruits like tomato, cucumber and bell peppers cannot be combined with sweet fruits but can be combined with each other. Bananas are mildly mucus forming so it's not a good idea to eat a lot of bananas at a time. One or two is usually enough. Bananas are fattening, so you have to watch how many you eat because they have a lot of calories. Bananas are a very sweet, non-juicy fruit and they can drain minerals from your teeth, so they are best eaten in moderation.

The same goes for dates, which are very sweet and can de-mineralize your teeth from the excess sugar. Dried fruits like raisins and dried bananas are very sweet and can cause tooth decay.

A serious case of gas and indigestion can occur by eating fruits after eating vegetables or eating too soon after the last meal. The stomach needs to be empty before eating again. Sweet fruits blended together in a smoothie or eaten with vegetables like lettuce or celery can cause indigestion because you are digesting two different types of foods. The exception to this is apples which can be eaten with celery or sliced into a vegetable salad.

This way of eating doesn't get boring because high quality tree and vine ripened fruit is so satisfying. Living fruit brings you to LIFE.

Be careful of orange juice and pineapples due to their high acid content. Perfectly ripe yellow and white pineapple are sweet and not overly acidic. Pineapple eaten whole in excess, even when perfectly ripe, can eat away at your mouth giving you sores and also eat away at the enamel of your teeth.

Papaya and bananas are available year round in the tropics and sub-tropics.

Whole carob pods and carob powder mixed with bananas are excellent mineral supplements on a diet high in fruits. Raw carob powder is available year round and can be combined with banana to make mineral rich treats. Shape the carob-banana dough into brownies, cake or cookies as desired. A moist texture can be had using more banana and a little purified water. Natural vanilla powder adds flavor.

FRUIT: VITAMIN RICH

After going on a transition diet, you can thrive on nothing but non-fatty, sweet, juicy fruit (fig, papaya, melon etc.) and non-sweet fruit (tomato, cucumber, bell pepper), green leafy vegetables, root vegetables, tender greens, grasses, herbs and raw cultured milk.

Healthy, high quality fruits grown on mineral-rich soil are high in mineral and vitamin content and thus able to support a higher, more vital level of health and well-being. The fruit and vegetable diet can be adapted to your particular produce supply, climate and lifestyle.

You can enjoy excellent health on a mucusless/lean diet. If you are eating one fruit meal per day and drinking fruit juice you are consuming quite enough fruit to achieve radiant health. The ideal would be to have access to mineralized fruits, vegetables and grass-fed, cultured milk, an ideal climate and a low-stress, country lifestyle.

There are so many fruits to choose from that one will never lack variety in the diet. These include all the ideal tree and vine fruits such as apple, orange, grape, plum, apricot, cherry, peach, nectarine, berries, sweet melons, banana, cherimoya, mango and all the botanic plant fruits like tomato, cucumber, bell pepper, squash, zucchini, okra and eggplant.

Fresh ripe fruit in season like tree-ripened mangos or fresh figs or sweet cherimoyas or peaches are the true food of humans with botanic fruits, vegetables, herbs and cultured milk as secondary supportive foods.

The king of fruits is the apple with many varieties. The queen of fruit is the mango from the warm tropics. Grapes have to be high on the list since they are mentioned in the Bible many times. Grapes need a warm summer climate to thrive.

Figs are another most celestial fruit. Berries, when vine ripened, are not sour but sweet and delicious. Plums when tree ripened on a warm summer day cannot be forgotten, nor sweet nectarines or peaches. What about sweet watermelon on a hot summer day?

Did we forget apricots grown to perfection without irrigation, like little mangos and cherries so fulfilling and warming with their bright red color. Fruits inspire the virtues of courage, compassion, creativity and joy because they are chock full of vital, life energy found in their enzymes, hormones, vitamins and other phyto-chemicals. Food becomes the consumer and you are mentally what you eat physically.

THE MAXIMUM TEMPERATURE WE CAN HEAT FOOD AND STILL CLAIM IT'S A LIVING FOOD

If the food is too hot to touch that means that some enzymes are being destroyed.

Most living food enthusiasts know 118 degrees °F (Fahrenheit) as the top limit of heating food. Dr. John Whitaker, from U.C. Davis, says that most enzymes will not become completely inactive until food temperatures exceed 140 °F to 158 °F in a wet state.

Dr. Edward Howell (1985) in his book "Enzyme Nutrition" stated that prolonged temperatures over 118 °F will destroy enzymes, yet he also says in the book that the enzyme amylase can still convert starch to sugar at air temperatures up to 160 °F but will wear out after half an hour.

Dr. Howell also states that the optimum temperature for enzymes is between 45 °F to 140 °F So, to avoid any loss at all of food enzymes the food must not be heated above 118 °F, yet to minimize their loss, food could be heated to 140-158 °F.

According to Paul Kouchakoff M.D., a Swiss researcher at the Institute of Clinical Chemistry in Lausanne, Switzerland, water can be heated to 189 Fahrenheit (°F) or 87 Celsius (°C) without causing an increase in the number of white blood cells or leukocytosis (a raised white blood cell count or leukocyte count above the normal range in the blood) but if heated to 191 °F or 88 °C it causes the white blood cells to increase in order to clean, the now altered in structure, water.

For milk the critical temperature is 191 °F, for grains, tomatoes, cabbage and bananas it's 192 °F, pears and meat 194 °F, butter 196 °F, apples and oranges 197 °F, potatoes 200 °F, carrots, strawberries and figs 206 °F or 97 °C which is near the boiling temperature of 100 °C or 212 °F.

Boiling or steaming of food is done at a temperature of 212 °F.

Eating food cooked at this temperature causes the body to form excess lymphocytes or white blood cells. Lymphocytes use phagocytosis to engulf and consume, the now toxic, cooked food substance.

The smoke point or temperature at which olive oil starts smoking in the frying pan is 375 °F or 190 °C, so at these high temperatures you know the food is being damaged by high heat and will cause lymphocyte or white blood cell increase in the digestive tract and blood stream. Baking too is done at around 375 °F.

An electric slow cooker equipped with a warm temperature setting can cook at lower temperatures than steaming or boiling and thus prevent the formation of excess white blood cells (excess mucus).

A typical slow cooker operates at 80 °C (176 °F) on low, 90 °C (194 °F) on high and about 140 °F on the warm setting.

A kitchen thermometer is needed to check the actual food temperature. A slow cooker uses about the same amount of electricity as a light bulb, unlike the hotplate which guzzles energy.

If you must eat cooked food, combining raw foods high in food enzymes with low heat cooked foods (189-206 °F) would be useful in restoring the enzyme loss in the heated food. Thus you would have no white blood cell increase (mucus formation) and you would get more food enzymes eating raw salads with low heat, cooked food.

Some researchers have used Kouchakoff's experiments to say we can eat high temperature cooked foods if we eat them with 50% raw food. However, Kouchakoff specifically tells us that if we mix many different cooked foods, all with many different critical points, then eating raw food with them, it will not prevent the formation of increased white blood cells.

Most cooked food dishes have many cooked foods all mixed together. Raw food could neutralize cooked food if for example you only ate cooked squash and had a raw salad with grated carrot in it.

Grated carrot has a high critical point (206 F) so it would cancel the effect of the cooked squash and not produce the formation of white blood cells. During the transition, raw vegetables, with their high food enzyme content, are eaten with cooked vegetables and cooked starch to aid in digestion.

THE VALUE OF VEGETABLE JUICES

Vegetable juices help neutralize the waste products in the blood and thus make it easier to fast. Cucumber as a base with spinach, carrot, celery, tomato, cilantro, dandelion and parsley is a good "V-8" type, raw vegetable juice.

Cucumber juice is rich in silicon which is good for the skin (preventing wrinkles and aging) and the nails. It's also valuable for the kidneys providing minerals and cleansing for the renal filter system. Living, raw vegetable juices help remineralize the body. Celery juice is very good for the nervous system and removing calcium deposits due to its high organic sodium content. Dandelion leaf is easily found in most yards. It's high in calcium and regenerates the liver.

Most vegetable juices do not concentrate polyunsaturated fats, the exceptions being tomato juice which in a 100 gram or 3.5 oz serving has 1.0 mg omega-3 fatty acids and 23.0 mg omega-6 fatty acids and canned vegetable juice cocktail which has 1.0 mg omega-3 fatty acids and 36.0 mg omega-6 fatty acids. Canned V-8 vegetable juice has no unsaturated fats nor does wheatgrass juice or carrot juice.

The best way to extract fresh raw vegetable juice is to use a high quality vegetable juicer. A good choice is the Omega model 8003 Nutrition Center, white finish, the 8005 is the chrome model and is $30.00 more. It's good for extracting juice from pineapple, wheatgrass, parsley and leafy vegetables like spinach and lettuce. I purchased it online for $219.00 in 2003 (2013 price $229, chrome $259) which is a good price for this high quality type of juicer which crushes out the juice using a corkscrew gear at low speed to avoid oxidation of nutrients as occurs in centrifugal type juicers.

If you are very toxic, a short, one or two day vegetable juice fast will make it easier to fast. When you are more detoxified, try the one day, living water fast using both vegetable and fruit juices like orange, pineapple, apple and grape which will detoxify your body at a deeper level.

A longer fruit and vegetable juice fast is an advanced fast for those ready. Coconut water can also be used if you don't have a juicer. Avoid mineral or tap water because it's loaded with inorganic minerals which lodge in the joints creating stiffness. Living water from fruits and vegetables is the best drink for fasting and normal eating.

LIST OF MUCUS FORMING
AND NON MUCUS FORMING FOODS

Mucus Forming Foods:
Eggs (very mucus forming)
White/Brown Rice, Corn and other Cooked Grains, Pasta, Noodles
Bread, Pastry, Cake, Pie, Cookies, Doughnuts
Olive Oil, All Vegetable Oils Including Cold Pressed
Nuts, Coconut (Hard and Jelly), Seeds (Seed Cheese), Beans,
Soy (Tempeh, Miso, Tofu, Soy Sauce, Soy Meat, Soy Yogurt)
Bread (Rye crisp and Well Toasted Bread is less mucus forming)
Meat, Fish, Seafood, Fowl (very acidic)
Avocado, Durian
Cooked Potato
Pasteurized, Grain-Fed, Hard and Soft Cheeses
Pasteurized, Grain-Fed, Yogurt
Pasteurized, Grain-Fed, Cottage Cheese
Pasteurized, Grain-Fed, Butter
(Pasture-Raised, Raw Dairy Products; Cheese, Cottage Cheese, Yo-
gurt, Butter, Sour Cream are generally non mucus forming, they can
form the good, clear to white mucus which protects the mucus mem-
branes but not the green or yellow mucus which the body gets rid of
during colds)
Sweet Banana (mildly mucus forming in excess)
Starchy or Cooked Green Bananas (mildly mucus forming)
Cooked Cauliflower (mildly mucus forming)

Non Mucus Forming Foods:
All Tree, Vine, Bush and Plant Fruits
Ideal Juicy Sweet Fruits: Apple, Mango, Strawberries, Blackberries,
Cherries, Fig, Peach, Plum, Apricot, Papaya, Grapes, Orange, Manda-
rin, Cherimoya, Nectarine, Melons
Sweet Fruits: Bananas, Carob powder/pod, Dates, Raisins, Dried
Fruit
Non Sweet, Botanic or Vegetable Fruits: Tomatoes, Cucumbers, Bell
Peppers
All Green, Starchless Vegetables: Lettuce, Spinach, Celery, Cabbage,
Kale, Carrot, Beet, Radish, Dandelion, Parsley, Wheat Grass
Starchy Vegetables (cooked): Broccoli (can be eaten raw), Winter
Squash, Summer Squash, Zucchini, Eggplant (Aubergine), Artichoke,
String Beans, Okra

THE TRANSITION DIET
QUICK START-UP PROGRAM

The following actions will get you started quickly on the transition diet in order to start reaping the benefits of a clean system.

1. REDUCE CONGESTING, MUCUS FORMING FOODS THAT CLOG YOU UP AND SLOW YOU DOWN.

Eat one meat-free day per week to start, then add more days when you are ready. Choose organic, grass-fed beef, lamb and pork, low mercury fish and organic, free-range chicken and turkey. Marinated tempeh soy meat and raw cheese are good meat alternatives.

Reduce fast foods, snack foods and grain products like breads, donuts, cookies and pastries. If you're vegetarian or vegan reduce or eliminate heavy, mucus forming soybean products (tofu, soy milk, soy yogurt), beans, nuts, seeds, bread and eggs. For protein and fat use homemade, raw milk yogurt, mayonnaise, natural cheese, green peas, spirulina, olive oil, olives, sour cream, butter and coconut oil.

2. START EATING TWO BIG MEALS A DAY.

Eating many small meals throughout the day just clogs you up and slows you down.

Instead drink delicious juices for breakfast like fresh made orange juice or pineapple juice or a cucumber, carrot, tomato, celery, parsley, spinach mix. Juice filtered through a strainer, contains no fiber that can start the digestive process, allowing you to fast and cleanse without feeling discomfort and weakness. Juice will neutralize toxins, provide minerals, vitamins and natural plant sugar giving you a burst of energy.

Get a good juicer like the Omega chrome finished juicer (around $259) to make the task of juicing easier. If you get weak or hungry eat another meal, but try to adapt to two big meals per day if possible.

For lunch have a salad (dressed with protein and fat), cooked vegetables and a cooked starch. It's possible to eat just twice a day if you have high quality juices for breakfast which allows you to fast until the mid-day vegetable meal. If this doesn't work then eat a big meal in the morning and at mid-day and have juice, soup or if needed some fruit in the evening.

3. START EATING A BIG LETTUCE SALAD, STEAMED VEG-ETABLES AND COOKED POTATOES, BROWN RICE (WHOLE GRAIN) OR HIGH FIBER RYE CRISPBREAD AS THE STAPLES OF YOUR DIET.

Salad, cooked vegetables (broccoli, string beans, cabbage, cauliflower) and cooked potatoes or brown rice can be prepared in many delicious ways using herbs and sauces. Check out the many recipe ideas in the recipe section of this book.

The "vegetable broom" (the fiber in salads and cooked vegetables) will help sweep out the whole digestive tract quickly, making you feel like a brand new person. Flexitarians, also called semi-vegetarians (reduced meat diet) can eat their meat with the salad and vegetables, not the cooked starch to aid digestion.

4. DO A 40 HOUR FAST.

Regular, consistent, short fasts are the best way to slowly detox your body without losing your vital energy reserves. A long fast when just starting the transition will do more harm than good because of the toxic overload of the eliminative organs.

To do a 40 hour fast eat dinner, then skip breakfast, lunch and dinner the next day. Break the fast the next day at 9 a.m. to 12 noon by eating a vegetable meal if you are just starting the transition and a fruit meal if you are more advanced.

Upon rising the morning of the fast take the herbal laxative senna, available in bulk or teabags, to clean out the whole digestive tract. Using the bulk herb is more economical, just take a handful and boil it in two cups of filtered water, then simmer at low heat until it's down to one half cup. Filter this mixture using a metal or plastic sieve, then drink it. In three to six hours your bowels will move which empties any toxic matter in the large intestine. This makes it easier to fast because the bloodstream is not being re-contaminated by stored waste trapped in the colon.

Drink juices filtered with a sieve throughout the fast. Bottled apple juice can be used when just starting the transition because it will cleanse the body less than living, raw juices. Watermelon or other melons can be juiced in your mouth by chewing the pulp, swallowing the liquid then spitting out all the fiber and seeds. Orange juice is best used in moderation, due to its acidity. Vegetable juices like a cucumber, tomato, celery, carrot, spinach, parsley blend is delicious. Filter it three times, the third time grate 3 cloves of garlic in the sieve. Heat until warm or hot, but not scalding hot or boiling.

5. START ENJOYING THE BENEFITS OF A CLEAN, PROPERLY FED BODY.

Enjoy the transition! Know that you are slowly cleaning out your body and replacing the mucus and toxins with organic, living water, minerals, vitamins, hormones, phytonutrients, natural fatty acids and protein. These are the best building blocks available for creating a strong, healthy body.

Immediately you will begin to feel the difference as you let go of the sticky mucus and toxic matter in your intestines and cellular spaces. You are on your way to ideal health.

6. START A SMALL SALAD GARDEN SO YOU CAN ENJOY THE BENEFITS OF FRESH PRODUCE PICKED THE SAME DAY.

It's so much fun watching the plants grow and then picking them fresh at the peak of maturity, ensuring the best tasting produce possible. Lettuce, tomatoes, cucumbers, carrots, beets, kale, kohlrabi, radishes and onions are easy to grow from seed.

You could also plant a few fruit trees, berry plants and grapes for the future. Berries will start producing in a year, grapes in two or three years and grafted trees need two or more years usually.

MINERALS, VITAMINS AND
ESSENTIAL FATS

RE-MINERALIZING THE BODY

The adult body contains approximately 1,200 grams or 2.65 pounds of calcium, of which approximately 99% is present in the skeleton and teeth.

The other 1% of body calcium is found in extracellular fluids, intracellular structures and cell membranes. Non-skeletal calcium plays an essential role in such vital functions as nerve conduction, muscle contraction, blood clotting and membrane permeability.

Double Noble Laureate Dr. Linus Pauling said: "One could trace every sickness, every disease and every ailment to a mineral deficiency." Dentist Dr. Melvin Page found if he could get his patient's calcium/phosphorus ratio to be 10 to 4 or 2.5 times more calcium than phosphorus, their tooth decay would stop.

Calcium is a substance that is necessary for healthy bones. Dairy products are one of the best sources of dietary calcium. In fact, the American diet depends on dairy products for about 75 percent of its calcium. Calcium salts are calcium in an inorganic, metallic form that is bound to chemical salts. Since these forms are inorganic the body does not readily absorb these salts and utilize them efficiently. Yet, their low cost makes them a common choice for formulating products.

The most common calcium supplement found is calcium carbonate, from ground limestone or oyster shell, or calcium phosphate and calcium lactate. Others include calcium citrate, calcium aspartate, calcium orotate and calcium gluconate. These minerals are often too large to pass through the intestinal walls intact so they must be restructured for absorption.

Amino acid chelated calcium is a calcium molecule bound by two amino acids. This process involved wrapping amino acids or protein around metallic minerals to help the body metabolize them. Supplement manufacturers claim that chelated minerals are organic, just as minerals are found in plants. Chelation did help the problem because the added dissolvers did increase the assimilation to about 40% from 8% for metallic minerals. However, chelated or not, the fact remains, they're still metallic minerals and we are designed to use minerals derived from vegetation and fruits.

The U.S. National Academy of Sciences recommends (RDI or

Reference Daily Intake which replaces the RDA) 1,200 mg calcium per day for someone over 50 and 1,000 mg for those 19 to 50. It's interesting to note that at the time of our most rapid growth of our bones, which is the first six months of our life, we live on mother's milk which only contains 33 mg calcium per 100 grams.

The greatest concern on a fruit and vegetable based diet is that one will develop tooth decay and osteoporosis due to a low mineral intake. Eating green, unripe fruit, citrus especially, but also any fruit which is too acid (like pineapples or pomegranates) can etch away at the tooth enamel.

Also it's important not to cut oranges or other citrus fruits into wedges and then bite into them, since this wears away the enamel by contact. Honey, raw cane sugar, brown sugar, white sugar, agave syrup, maple syrup, rice syrup and dried fruit all drain the mineral reserves of the body and can cause tooth decay.

Given a healthy diet and moderate exercise, large-boned animals like cows and horses do not suffer from osteoporosis, even though they don't have a high calcium intake.

How do chickens manage to produce all the internal calcium they need to make egg shells day after day? The horse and cow biologically transmute chlorophyll rich grass which is high in magnesium into calcium and the chicken eat mica which is silica and transmute it to calcium. We too can transmute minerals but not to the extent that these animals can and thus we must consume grass-fed, raw dairy products.

Now to the other extreme an excess intake of calcium may cause muscle spasms, unwanted deposits such as bone spurs or plaque on the walls of blood vessels or in the kidneys, heart, and liver and may increase the risk of cancer, kidney stones, depression and heart arrhythmia.

Americans consume dairy products and calcium supplements at one of the highest rates in the world, yet they have one of the highest rates of osteoporosis in the world. About 85%-90% of American dairy products come from grain-fed, hormone-injected, corral-kept cows which results in dairy products that lack vitamin A, D, E and K, the fat solubles. Green grass is what gives milk its high vitamin A, D, E and K content. Without these fat soluble vitamins the body can't absorb calcium. Calcium supplements in the inorganic form like calcium carbonate are poorly absorbed compared to natural, organic, food derived calcium as found in grass-fed, dairy products.

The ideal calcium-phosphorus ratio is 2 to 1, close to the proportion found in human milk. The higher the phosphorus content of the food, the more calcium is excreted in the urine, leading to a loss of calcium which can cause tooth decay, toothache, bone weakening and nervous problems.

The calcium-phosphorus ratio of foods like sirloin steak (2 mg calcium to 229 mg phosphorus), corn (calcium 10 mg to 120 mg phosphorus) and soy burgers (29 mg calcium to 344 mg phosphorus) makes them rob calcium from the teeth and bones.

An excellent source of calcium so you can have strong, hard teeth is Swiss cheese. It's a "holy cheese" not because it has holes in it, but because it's such a great source of calcium, vitamin D, A and K and vitamin B-12. Lactobacillus bacteria start the Swiss cheese cultivation process, which means the cheese contains living, active Lactobacillus bacteria in it. It's non mucus forming using moderate amounts.

A good source of minerals to keep the teeth and bones healthy are carob powder and carob powder mixed with bananas (can be mixed with bananas to form brownies or it can be made into a smoothie with bananas and papaya), dark leafy green vegetables like spinach, dandelion and bibb lettuce, papayas and raw cheese, raw milk yogurt and raw milk cottage cheese (use natural, grass-fed, pasteurized dairy products if you are unable to find raw milk cheese, yogurt and cottage cheese).

A good calcium supplement is Garden of Life brand Raw Calcium because it's high also in magnesium and has vitamin D to aid absorption. A good silicon supplement is Flora brand silica capsules made by the Kervran method. Kelp can be taken in tablet form. Dulse, a red colored, good-tasting seaweed can be eaten whole, flaked, powdered, as a liquid extract or in tablets.

Seaweed needs to be washed thoroughly in order to remove the excess salt content, then it can be soaked in purified water. It will expand many times its size. Season with a little lemon and lime juice. Nori and nori flakes are also mineral rich sea vegetable products. Maine Coast Sea Vegetables sells sea vegetables and they are certified organic and, after the Japanese nuclear disaster, radiation free.

Be very careful about foods that drain calcium from your teeth and bones. Highly acidic fruits like pineapples and pineapple juice (especially greenish, not fully ripe pineapples) and citrus fruits (especially unripe, greenish tinged citrus fruits), including oranges, mandarin oranges, tangerines, tangelos, grapefruit, lemons and limes will drain calcium from your body because the body will neutralize the acid by taking calcium from the teeth and bones.

Even if the citrus and pineapples are completely ripe they are highly acidic. The teeth are the first to be drawn on because they are not part of the structure of the body.

Dried fruit like raisins, prunes, dried pineapple and dried bananas are very concentrated in sugar and that tends to draw calcium out the body. They are also very sticky and the sugar sticks to the teeth which the bacteria immediately use and produce an acid by-product which etches away at the teeth.

LIST OF MINERAL RICH
FRUITS AND VEGETABLES

High Magnesium Fruits (all figures in milligrams or mg per 100 grams)
Date 58
Carob 54
Banana 33
Blackberry and black raspberry 30
Granadilla 29
Fig and red raspberry 20
High Magnesium Vegetables
Kelp 760
Spinach 88
Swiss chard 65
Turnip greens 58
Collards 57
Parsley and Okra 41
Kale and Kohlrabi 37
Fresh green pea 35
Potato with skin 34

High Silicon Fruits
Strawberry 783
Cherry 311
Apricot 280
Tomato 175
Watermelon 160
Apple 142
Banana 80
Plum 68
Grapes 60
High Silicon Vegetables
Lettuce, Boston, Bibb 2400
Iceberg Lettuce 1464
Asparagus 950
Spinach 810
Cucumber 800
Artichoke, Globe 530
Lettuce Cos, Romaine 530
Celery 430
Cauliflower 337
Kohlrabi 205

High Potassium Fruits
Tamarind 781
Date 648
Black currant 372
Banana 370
Granadilla 348
Persimmon, American 310
Elderberry 300
Damson plum 299
Nectarine 294
Guava 289
High Potassium Vegetables
Dulse 8060
Kelp 5273
Parsley 727
Spinach 470
Artichoke, Globe 430
Potato with skin 407
Broccoli 382

High Iron Fruits
Date 3.0
Carob 2.94
Tamarind 2.8
Persimmon 2.5
Granadilla 1.6
Elderberry 1.6
Carambola 1.5
Loganberry, Longan 1.2
Roseapple 1.2
High Iron Vegetables
Dulse 150
Kelp 100
Parsley 6.2
Purslane leaves 3.5
Jerusalem artichoke 3.4
Spinach 3.1
Kale leaves 2.7
Lettuce Boston Bibb 2.0
Lettuce Cos Romaine 1.4

High Calcium Fruits
Carob flour 348
Tamarind 74
Kumquat 63
Lemon with peel 61
Black currant 60
Date 59
Orange peeled 41
Tangerine 40
Sapote 39
Fig 35
High Calcium Vegetables
Kelp 1093
Collard greens 250
Kale 249
Parsley 203
Broccoli and Purslane 103
Spinach 99
Swiss chard 88

Good mineral sources of calcium are farmer's cheese, cottage cheese, raw yogurt, carob powder mashed with banana and papaya, vegetable juice (cucumber, carrot, celery, spinach, tomato, parsley), food source and food grown minerals, kelp powder and dulse leaves from known pollution and radiation free sources like Maine Coast Sea Vegetables.

VITAMINS AND MINERALS: THE CURRENT RECOMMENDED AMOUNTS

Dietary Reference Intakes (DRI) are the most recent set of dietary recommendations established by the Food and Nutrition Board of the Institute of Medicine (1997-2001). They replace the RDAs or Recommended Daily Allowance and may be the basis for eventually updating the RDIs.

The Reference Daily Intake (RDI) is the value established by the Food and Drug Administration for use in food labeling. It was based initially on the highest 1968 RDA for each nutrient, to assure that needs were met for all age groups. The DRIs may be the basis for eventually updating the RDIs.

Nutrients are now assigned either an Estimated Average Requirement (EAR) and Recommended Daily Allowance (RDA) or an Adequate Intake (AI) value for each life stage category. Most nutrients also have a Tolerable Upper Intake Level (UL) to prevent the risk of adverse effects from excessive nutrient intakes.

The new RDAs and AIs serve as intake goals. The current DRIs are divided into the groups; infants, children, males, females, pregnancy and lactating with various age groups within each group. The website of the USDA Food and Nutrition Information Center can be accessed for your specific group.

The following are my DRIs (male age 51-70) which are very similar to other adult groups: Minerals: Calcium 1000 mg, Iron 8 mg, Phosphorus 700 mg, Iodine 150 mcg, Magnesium 420 mg, Zinc 11 mg, Selenium 55 mcg, Copper 0.9 mg, Manganese 2.3 mg, Chromium 30 mcg, Molybdenum 45 mcg.

The current DRIs for vitamins (male age 51-70) are: Vitamin A 900 mcg (3000 IU), Vitamin C 90 mg, Vitamin D 15 mcg (600 IU) (Vitamin D is a hormone your body makes when exposed to the sun. You can get some of what you need if you live in the sub-tropics or tropics, the rest is provided by grass-fed dairy products), Vitamin E 15 mg (15 mg is defined as the equivalent of 22 IU of natural vitamin E or 33 IU of synthetic vitamin E.), Vitamin K 120 mcg, Thiamin 1.2 mg, Riboflavin 1.3 mg, Niacin 16 mg, Vitamin B-6 1.7 mg, Folate 400 mcg from food, 200 mcg synthetic, Vitamin B-12 2.4 mcg (It is recommended that people over 50 meet the B-12 recommendation through fortified foods or supplements, to improve bioavailability), Biotin 30 mcg, Pantothenic acid 5 mg, Choline 550 mg, omega-3 1.6 gm/day, omega-6 14 gms/day.

To find your particular DRIs go to the USDA Food and Nutrition Information Center online.

Most people don't go around counting their daily vitamin and mineral intake. Take a quality multivitamin/mineral supplement if you want to be sure.

Self Magazine's NutritionData website has a free program that will analyze your diet. Most people eat the same foods day after day, so to get a good idea of how close your diet comes to the DRIs, it's worth the effort to check out your diet using their free online program. Google NutritionData to find out if you are getting enough vitamins and minerals.

VITAMIN B-12

"All of the Vitamin B-12 in the world ultimately comes from bacteria. Neither plants nor animals can synthesize it.", says Virginia Messina, MPH, RD, author of *The Vegetarian Way*. The human mouth and the upper and lower intestine all contain bacteria that produce B-12.

In some cases, the symptoms of vitamin B12 deficiency can be vague, take years to develop, or may not be noticeable immediately. Some symptoms of vitamin B12 deficiency are due to a decreased production of red blood cells, which are necessary to carry vital oxygen to the body's cells and tissues.

Symptoms of vitamin B12 deficiency can affect the gastrointestinal tract, the nervous system, and the cardiovascular system. Symptoms of vitamin B12 deficiency include: chest pain or heart palpitations, confusion, memory loss or dementia, constipation, depression, developmental delays and failure to thrive, dizziness, trouble maintaining balance, fainting, fatigue or weakness, numbness or coldness of hands and feet, pale skin or jaundice (yellowing of skin and eyes), poor appetite, shortness of breath, sore mouth and tongue and weight loss.

Most people with Vitamin B-12 deficiencies or pernicious anemia are not vegans and is due to lack of intrinsic factor, parasites or chemicals that destroy B-12.

In India the vegans (no animal foods) don't get B-12 deficiency because the produce is unwashed and contaminated with human and animal manure bacteria, which provides all the B-12 that they need.

Joel Robbins, D.C., N.D. says bananas, Concord grapes and plums have vitamin B-12, which is due to the bacteria they harbor.

Most produce is washed excessively these days so it wouldn't hurt to take a good quality multi-vitamin supplement just to make sure you're getting all your vitamins, especially if you've been vegan for a long period of time.

Garden of Life, New Chapter and Megafood food grown nutrients are good choices. Or one can buy the methyl form of vitamin B-12, which is superior to the cyano form, as an individual supplement.

One cup of whole milk yogurt has .91 mcg. of B-12, so 3 cups daily will provide 2.73 mcg. which is more than the DRI of 2.4 mcg.

Beneficial bacteria manufacture B vitamins and amino acids and help us absorb food and minerals. Acidophilus and bifidobacterium are two examples of beneficial bacteria. The growth of good bacteria helps to crowd out disease causing bacteria such as E. coli and Clostridia which convert chemicals to carcinogens and also create free radicals.

Good bacteria produce short-chain fatty acids (SCFA) which make the colon slightly acidic which prevents the growth of harmful bacteria and aids in the absorption of calcium and magnesium.

The trillion bacteria cells in our bodies outnumber our own cells by ten times and weigh about 3 pounds. We tend to think of bacteria as being all harmful but we need their symbiotic help to live. The bacteria in our gut are crucial for our survival. Good gut bacteria help our immune system fight off bad bacteria from infecting our bio-sphere.

Homemade, raw milk yogurt and salt-free, raw sauerkraut (fermented green cabbage) will help keep the colon filled with good bacteria.

The great hygiene and sanitation reform in the United States did a lot of good in removing some infectious diseases by improving poor sewage disposal and treatment, garbage collection, cleanliness in food processing and clean drinking water. Bacteriology made us aware of bacterial contamination but excessive hygiene cuts us off from our bacterial vitamin sources as found in unwashed produce.

KEYS TO HEALING YOUR TEETH: VITAMIN K2 MK-4, THE CALCIUM/PHOSPHORUS RATIO AND AVOIDING EXCESSIVE FRUIT ACIDS AND SUGARS

Living on just fruit can damage your teeth permanently. Citrus, especially unripe citrus, orange juice, pineapples and pineapple juice and unripe mangos are all notorious for damaging your teeth. Strict, fruit only fruitarianism and strict, raw veganism can damage your teeth in the long run because these diets lack vitamin K2 MK-4, which is only found in animal products. Tom Sanders, a professor in nutrition and dietetics at King's College, London, studied tooth decay in youngsters and found that those from vegan or "fruitarian" families, who eat only fruit, often had the worst teeth.

Dr. Weston Price used butter oil (clarified butter or ghee) and cod liver oil to reverse dental caries. The dentin remineralized and sealed the dental decay with a glassy finish. In the numerous butter samples tested, **"Activator X"** was present only when the animals were eating rapidly growing green grass occurring in high rainfall periods. Price found the highest concentrations of **Activator-X** in the milk of several species, varying with the nutrition of the animal."

Dr. Price used butter oil and cod liver oil to heal teeth, so the elusive **Activator-X** factor, which he could not identify, was the animal derived vitamin K2 MK-4 not the bacteria/plant derived MK-7 form. The MK-7 form of K2 can be produced by bacterial fermentation, natto is the highest source with sauerkraut being a minor source. MK-4 is the type that mammals synthesize for themselves. Instead of cod liver oil vegetarians can use dark yellow butter, butter oil, grass-fed cheese and yogurt. In cases of serious tooth decay you can buy a complete form of K-2 like Life Extension's Super K w/ Advanced K2 Complex or Vitacost's Ultra Vitamin K with Advanced K2 Complex which contains MK-4, Mk-7 and K1.

Dr. Holly Roberts D.O., a board certified Obstetrician/Gynecologist and author of *Your Vegetarian Pregnancy* says, "Calcium deficiency can occur, not only if your diet is low in calcium, but also if your diet is high in phosphorus. The ratio of calcium to phosphorus in your bones is 2.5 to 1. If your diet includes higher levels of calcium than phosphorus, it is more likely that you will maintain this healthy ratio and healthy bones. To do this, it is best if you maintain a ratio of phosphorous to calcium within your diet of 1:1. The diet of many Americans contains a phosphorous-to-calcium ratio of 4:1. Calcium is a positive ion, which means it will bind with negative ions. Foods that contain phosphorus form negative ions. So if you have excess phosphorus in your diet, it will bind calcium to it and you will excrete both of these minerals. If such a situation develops, you may actually lose more calcium than you took in, and you will deplete the calcium stored in your bones (and teeth)." Sprouted wheat (raw, Essene bread) has 7 times more phosphorus than calcium or a Calcium to Phosphorus ratio of 1/7 (28 mg Ca/200 mg P per 100 grams) which will pull calcium from the teeth and bones.

It is widely recognized that sugar can cause tooth decay, the threat posed by acids, which strip away tooth enamel, is less well-known. A The British Dental Association (BDA) spokesman said: "Apples have a high acidity content and one of the things we are concerned about is erosion. Tooth decay is on the decline because of the introduction of fluoride in water and improved oral health. But erosion is becoming a real problem and something we are trying to raise awareness of. Research shows that dental erosion in adults due to diet is usually a result of excessive consumption of fruits and fruit juices." Parents should only give fruit juice to their children if it was heavily diluted, said the spokesman. The British Dental Association suggests that those seeking a snack between meals should eat cheese, despite its high fat content, because it neutralizes the acidity that can attack tooth enamel.

Brushing your teeth right after eating an apple does more harm than good, because enamel softened by the acid attack is scrubbed away by the toothbrush. Wait at least half an hour before brushing. Better to rinse with baking soda right after eating fruit and not brush.

Fruit teas can damage tooth enamel. Researchers at the University Dental Hospital of Manchester placed extracted teeth in three different liquids; a blackcurrant, ginseng and vanilla herbal tea, traditional tea and water. After 14 days the herbal tea had dissolved a layer of enamel from the tooth several millimeters thick.

Dextrose or dextrorotatory glucose is also called grape sugar. According to Dr. Richard Johnson, author of *The Sugar Fix*, dextrose, which is pure powdered glucose, has no effect on insulin resistance. The problem with dextrose, maltodextrin and table sugar is that they are chemically produced isolates of naturally occurring sugars and need to be avoided in order to heal cavities. Dextrose will rot your teeth just like sugar will.

Xylitol held much hope in preventing cavities and not causing insulin resistance. The problem is that it's toxic to animals. In lab tests, xylitol will kill a rat 50% of the time at a dosage of 16.5 grams of xylitol for every 1000 grams of rat. To kill a 100 gram rat, the rat only needs to consume, 1.65 grams of xylitol. A typical piece of xylitol gum contains .7 to 1 gram of xylitol or about half the amount needed to kill a rat.

Xylitol is also known to be deadly to dogs and other animals. Why should this product be allowed if it's known to be toxic to animals? The FDA or Food and Drug Administration did not put it on the GRAS or Generally Recognized As Safe list. It is only approved for cosmetic use like in toothpaste and gum.

In order to produce xylitol a highly complex process is used to produce it including hydrogenation using powdered nickel-aluminium alloy, plus further processing using acetic acid and ethanol. Processed, extracted sugar of all kinds is bad for your health and your teeth, especially because they deplete the minerals chromium, zinc, magnesium and manganese. There are too many risk factors involved with eating xylitol so it's best to stick to moderate use of natural sweeteners like stevia and unheated, raw honey.

Stevia has been used by humans for hundreds of years and by diabetic patients in Japan for decades. In the early 1970s, Japan began cultivating stevia as an alternative to artificial sweeteners such as cyclamate and saccharin, which were suspected carcinogens. Japan consumes more stevia than any other country, with stevia accounting for 40% of their sweetener market. Stevia may induce insulin secretion, but it also increases insulin sensitivity, reduces blood glucose and does not increase appetite. Stevia may also inhibit the growth of the bacteria that cause tooth decay and gum disease. It's best to use the whole dried leaf stevia for use in sun teas and boiled tea or a powdered version of the dried leaf or a water extract of the whole leaf. Highly processed extracts of stevia are not natural and may cause problems.

MEGADOSE VITAMIN C

Dr. Fred Klenner used Vitamin C in the form of sodium ascorbate intravenously for carbon monoxide poisoning, barbiturate poisoning and snakebites. An adult male came to his office complaining of severe chest pain and the inability to take a deep breath. He said he had been "stung" or "bitten" 10 minutes earlier. He begged for help saying he was dying. He was becoming cyanotic (blue or livid skin from lack of oxygen). Twelve grams of vitamin C was quickly pulled into a 50 c.c. syringe and with a 20 gauge needle was given intravenously as fast as the plunger could be pushed. Even before the injection was completed, he exclaimed, "Thank God". The poison had been neutralized that rapidly. He was sent home to locate the "culprit". Duke University identified it as the Puss Caterpillar. If not for vitamin C this individual would have died from shock and asphyxiation.

Dr. Cathcart discovered that the sicker a patient is, the more vitamin C they can tolerate. Here is how he describes it: "In 1969, I discovered that the amount of ascorbic acid (not ascorbate, pure ascorbic acid) tolerated orally without loosening of stools (a benign diarrhea) was somewhat proportional to the free radical toxicity of the condition being treated. The sicker a person was, the more ascorbic acid they would tolerate orally without it causing diarrhea. A person with an otherwise normal GI tract, when they were well, would tolerate 5 to 15 grams of ascorbic acid orally in divided doses without diarrhea. With a mild cold 30 to 60 grams; with a bad cold, 100 grams; with a flu, 150 grams; and with mononucleosis, viral pneumonia, etc. 200 grams or more of ascorbic acid would be tolerated orally without diarrhea. The process of finding what dose will cause diarrhea and will eliminate the acute symptoms, I call titrating to bowel tolerance. If you have a 100-gram cold and the patient is taking roughly 100 grams a day, you will quickly eliminate perhaps 90% of the symptoms of the disease. But if you treat that same cold with 2 grams or even 20 grams a day, you won't see much happen." I met Dr. Cathcart in 1987 and he was treating AIDS with vitamin C. Dr. Cathcart treated AIDS patients with up to 200,000 milligrams (200 grams) of vitamin C a day and found that even advanced AIDS patients lived significantly longer and had far fewer symptoms.

The Vitamin C Foundation recommends L-ascorbic acid powder as the best, most powerful and fast acting form of vitamin C. Use a buffered form if you have trouble with the acidity. For intravenous or intramuscular injections Dr. Klenner used sodium ascorbate which is ascorbic acid buffered with sodium bicarbonate. Linus Pauling used buffered ascorbic acid (3.5 pH for pure ascorbic acid), using sodium bicarbonate (baking soda). Take 1 heaping teaspoon (5,000 mg) Vitamin C Crystals (l-ascorbic acid crystals) with one-half teaspoon (2,500 mg) of baking soda (sodium bicarbonate), mixed in an 8 ounce glass of juice. Or just buy sodium ascorbate which is about the same price.

SALT

The US government has lowered their sodium recommendations and is now recommending that people get 1,500 milligrams of sodium a day, about a heaping teaspoon, down from the current recommendation of 2,400 milligrams. According to the Institute of Medicine's report, this is the amount needed by healthy 19 to 50 year old adults to replace the amount lost each day through sweat while taking in an adequate diet. They set the "tolerable upper intake level" for salt at 5,800 milligrams a day, but note that over 95 percent of American men and 75 percent of American women regularly consume more than that.

The DRI (dietary reference intake) adequate intake for sodium is 1,500 mg (roughly half a teaspoon) and the maximum level is 2,300 mg a day if you're a healthy adult. You will need more in a very hot climate and if perspiring excessively.

Three-quarters of the salt Americans consume daily comes from processed and restaurant foods. Cutting back on processed/pre-packaged foods in your diet and using mostly fresh produce to make your food would drastically reduce the amount of salt you consume.

Explorers at sea for a long time or fisherman would cover their catch or food supply with salt in order to preserve it for at least a few days before they would return to the harbor.

Sodium chloride is a protoplasmic poison if used in excess. We are completely conditioned in the illusion of the necessity of salt. Yes, we need salt, but it's the "organic sodium" that is contained in fresh fruits and vegetables, especially celery, that we really need and not the inorganic sodium found in table salt and even Celtic or sea salt.

Food processors add salt to all their products in order to "hook" you on these denatured foods. Salt is addictive and it distorts your natural instincts and taste buds. Most people get far too much salt mostly from processed foods.

Mineral salt when it passes through a living plant, receives an accelerated atomic vibration, transforming it into vegetable salt. Mineral salt, in excess, is deposited like garbage inside the body especially in the arteries, provoking the dangerous disease called arteriosclerosis, high blood pressure and also blindness, deafness and dementia.

Vegetable salt that is found naturally in all vegetables and fruits is easily assimilated by the body. It purifies the blood and tissues, and lowers and normalizes blood pressure. Dr. Norman Walker wrote that organic sodium keeps inorganic calcium in solution in the body, which means if you have consumed a lot of bread, pasta, rice, and pastries the inorganic calcium that they contain will be slowly dislodged by drinking celery juice. Celery and celery juice have organic sodium which is not an inorganic earth metal but rather a plant created form of the element.

Dr. Max Gerson cured his and other people's migraine headaches by excluding all salt from their diet. My own personal experience is that when I used a lot of salt, dark lines formed underneath my eyes and the skin right below my eyes became wrinkled and dry. This indicates a strain on the kidneys according to Chinese medicine.

Sea salt is often marketed as a more natural and healthy alternative. The real differences between sea salt and table salt are in their taste but by weight, sea salt and table salt contain about the same amount of sodium chloride.

There are many alternatives to using salt like; lemon juice, grated fresh garlic, garlic powder, fresh chopped onion and onion powder. The commercial product Mrs. Dash has no salt, only dried herbs and spices.

There are a few studies touting salt's health benefits but if we look closer at the results and look at other studies showing that salt causes disease, we will arrive at the truth. Dr. Jan Staessen of the University of Leuven in Belgium and a group of researchers studied 3,681 people with no signs of high blood pressure or heart disease (Staessen et al, 2011). In the 8 years following the study's inception, there were 500% more deaths among the people who consumed the least amount of salt. What foods were let go of when they reduced their salt content? The people eating less salt may also be eating less dairy products which help prevent heart disease due to the vitamin K and natural saturated fat.

In Finland, when a reduced sodium replacement for table salt was used, they saw a 75 to 80% decrease in death from stroke and heart disease over 30 years according to a 2006 (Karppanen & Mervaala) study. This study shows that reducing inorganic sodium will reduce the death rate from stroke and heart disease, but what if all inorganic sodium was replaced? The death rate would fall even lower following the rules of logic.

Wright's salt is based on the reduced sodium salt used in Finland and consists of sodium chloride, potassium chloride, magnesium sulphate, lysine hydrochloride, silicon dioxide, zinc chloride, copper glycinate, selenium and potassium iodine. According to this study this is the healthiest salt you can consume, even healthier than Himalayan salt, Celtic salt and natural sea salt. A moderate amount of salt is ok during the transition because it helps neutralize any excess mucus and makes cooked starch more palatable. After the transition inorganic salt is no longer needed.

Raised blood pressure is the most important cause of heart disease, more important than smoking or elevated cholesterol, accounting for 62% of strokes and 49% of coronary heart disease (He & MacGregor, 2009). There is strong evidence that our current consumption of salt is the major factor increasing blood pressure and thereby cardiovascular disease.

A high salt diet may have direct harmful effects independent of its effect on BP (blood pressure), for example, increasing the risk of stroke, left ventricular hypertrophy and renal disease. Increasing evidence also suggests that salt intake is related to obesity through soft drink consumption, associated with renal stones and osteoporosis and is probably a major cause of stomach cancer.

In most developed countries, a reduction in salt intake can be achieved by a gradual and sustained reduction in the amount of salt added to food by the food industry. In other countries where most of the salt consumed comes from salt added during cooking or from sauces, a public health campaign is needed to encourage consumers to use less salt. Salt added to dairy products like cheese and butter is another problem to be addressed. A modest reduction in population salt intake worldwide will result in a major improvement in public health. Salt and also the reactive unsaturated fats like; cooking oil, trans fat partially hydrogenated oil, margarine (even non-trans fat) and even nuts, seeds, avocado and olive oil if eaten in excess, are the major causes of the cardio-vascular disease epidemic worldwide.

FOOD ENZYMES MUST BECOME
AS WELL KNOWN AS FOOD VITAMINS AND MINERALS

When any health professional talks about nutrition, they always include the vitamins and never remember that vitamins combine with proteins to create the metabolically active enzymes which run the processes of the body.

Vitamins are needed to make the metabolic enzymes function. Riboflavin or Vitamin B-2 works as a coenzyme in the metabolism of carbohydrates. Niacin or B-3 is a coenzyme that works to release energy from nutrients.

When you cut or burn your finger you anoint it with a piece of fresh aloe vera and it instantly eases the pain and starts the healing process. Aloe Vera contains 10 "food" or plant enzymes: Alkaline Phosphatase, Amylase, Carboxy-peptidase, Catalase, Cellulase, Lipase, Peroxidase and Bradykinase. Bradykinase helps to reduce excessive inflammation when applied to the skin topically and therefore reduces pain, whereas others help digest any dead tissues in wounds.

There's the proof from everyday practical living how food (plant) enzymes are healing agents. If eaten, aloe vera would help in the digestion of meals due to its containing active, living digestive enzymes which can help break down the meal.

You may ask, "Are the enzymes in the food we eat destroyed by the acids and enzymes in the stomach?" The answer is no, not all of them. Proof of this comes from Michael Gardner's study on the "Gastrointestinal Absorption of Intact Proteins" (1988) in which he states, "There is now irrefutable evidence that small amounts of intact peptides and proteins do enter the circulation under normal circumstances. Intact protein absorption must now be regarded as a normal physiological process in humans and animals... The concordance between results obtained by independent research using differentiated experiential approaches is now so strong that we cannot fail to accept that intact proteins and high molecular fragments thereof do cross the gastrointestinal tract in humans (both neonates and adults)."

This study shows that food enzymes, being proteins, are absorbed right through the stomach and intestinal walls. Between 12% and 70% of the proteolytic enzymes are absorbed into the blood stream intact from the gastro-intestinal tract. Approximately 6% of papain and 38% of bromelain taken orally is found to be active in the blood and lymph. Significant amounts of protease enzymes need to be taken because they are not 100% absorbed.

In 1992 in Germany, more than 1.4 million prescriptions of enzyme combinations were made with very few side effects reported. They are best taken one hour before or two hours after meals with water. Researchers have found special regions in the small intestine such as Peyer's patches where some of the largest enzymes are absorbed more rapidly than smaller enzyme molecules into the bloodstream.

The indigenous people of Central and South America have used the leaves and fruit of papaya and pineapples therapeutically for thousands of years. Enzymes were also used in Africa and India. The Bible mentions the use of figs for healing which are high in enzymes. The prophet Isaiah's use of figs and blessings to help heal King Hezekiah is enzyme therapy in Biblical times. In the Middle Ages the curative effect of many of the plants and fruits used was due to the proteases in them.

In terms of proteases or enzymes that digest proteins, bromelain from pineapple is better than papain from papaya and trypsin and chymotrypsin from animals for reducing swelling and edema.

Research with professional athletic teams shows that recovery time from injuries, swelling, and bruising is cut in half with the use of orally ingested proteolytic enzymes. Eating pineapple after a workout will help you recover faster. Bromelain is not as good as papain for breaking up antigen-antibody complexes, or for cell receptor modulation.

Protease function in the body are controlled by sequences of connecting enzymes. For example, at least five enzymes are needed for blood to clot, and five other enzymes are needed to dissolve the clotted blood. John Beard, a Scottish physician, in 1900 began to treat cancer patients with the enzymes of plants and the enzymes from the pancreases of freshly killed animals.

Max Wolf, an Australian-born, American-trained physician, is considered the father of systemic enzyme therapy. Dr. Wolf and Helen Benitez, a cell biologist developed proteolytic enzyme preparations for therapeutic uses, especially for the treatment of cancer. Wolf believed that premature aging is based on a deficiency of these enzymes. Wolf held that the key element of most aging processes are a disturbance in the physiological and regulatory mechanisms of the body.

He understood that enzymes are the keys to the proper functioning of the body's regulatory mechanisms, including the immune system. In 1960, enzyme combinations were introduced in Germany to help with the body's regulatory and immune system. Consult Gabriel Cousen's *Conscious Eating* (2000) for more information on food enzymes.

The Law of Adaptive Secretion of Digestive Enzymes states when you eat food enzymes in raw foods this spares the use and manufacture of your own enzymes. This law was scientifically proven in 1943 by Grossman, Greengard and Ivy; the body secretes no more digestive enzymes than are needed for the job. This law was confirmed by later researchers as well.

If you eat foods raw the food enzymes in the food will digest part of the food for you. The body can detect this and will secrete less enzymes in order to conserve its precious enzyme reserve.

Dr. Beazell (1941), in the American Journal of Physiology, showed that 60% of the complex carbohydrates, 30% of the protein and 10% of the fats are digested in the human food-enzyme stomach by the enzymes contained in raw food.

Cauliflower and broccoli are high in starch and are thus cooked to convert their starch to sugar to ease digestion during the transition. The presence of starch in raw cauliflower may cause gas and indigestion in some people.

Cabbage, broccoli and cauliflower can be eaten raw after the transition if it causes no indigestion. The starch in cauliflower when cooked is slightly mucus forming, but broccoli when cooked is not mucus forming at all. In general starchy vegetables are not mucus forming like cooked potato or cooked brown rice are, but their fiber does help somewhat in slowing down the elimination rate.

More than half of our production of protein (which is about 300 grams per day) is in making enzymes. Dr. Edward Howell M.D., to whom we owe our knowledge of food enzymes, has shown that cooked foods strain and over enlarge the pancreas from overwork.

If the food is cooked and enzyme-less the body will be forced to make and secrete more digestive enzymes and thus lose energy. It follows that the body will have more enzymes to repair itself and to prevent disease and aging if we eat fresh, uncooked, living foods.

Yet this is true only if a person goes through a lengthy, systematic detoxification. A toxic body cannot live on exclusively raw foods because the toxins stored in the body would be released too quickly, causing weakness, fever, cough, a runny nose, muscle aches or all the symptoms of a severe cold.

If one eats raw fruits that are high in food enzymes such as papaya, pineapple, mango, banana, figs and grapes one will really be saving their own digestive enzymes and thus receive the maximum benefit from eating raw foods.

Vegetables are low calorie foods which contain low amounts of food enzymes. This fact points to the truth that fruit is mankind's most important food, due to the high amounts of food enzymes they contain.

The enzyme maybe the spark of Life itself or Divinity within the human body. An enzyme gives life to the body. The life force in the air, also called prana by the East Indians and chi by the Chinese, is inspired with each breath. Sunlight contains energy that we absorb through our skin and eyes. All our social interactions nourish or deplete us. Our food and life energy sources are truly multi-dimensional.

THE AMAZING ENZYME:
THE SPARK OF LIFE

Enzymes are what moves the process we call life. Every bodily function such as the clotting of blood, the transmission of nerve signals, the sense of seeing, the contraction of the muscles, the process of thought are all made possible by enzymes. Enzymes run the process called bodily human life.

Each person has two types of enzymes in the body;
1. Metabolic (which run the processes of the body).
2. Digestive (which digest the food).

If your food is cooked its food enzymes are all destroyed. Thus, eating enzyme-less foods makes the body produce more digestive enzymes in order to compensate for the lack of food enzymes. Food enzymes help digest the food after it's eaten, therefore eating raw food high in enzymes saves the body from using its own.

To stop lowering one's enzyme level one must decrease enzyme loss by the creation of extra digestive enzymes in order to digest cooked food (it takes enzymes to make enzymes). Also we need to stop enzyme loss from adapting to external stressors such as excess heat or cold, poor personal hygiene, lack of sleep, air pollution, city traffic and noise, no sunlight, under or over exercise, exhausting trips, no social life, all of which can drain our enzyme bank.

The cooked food, enzyme-less diet forces the body to create high levels of digestive enzymes which greatly taxes the body's vital energy reserve. The most important measure for increasing your actual enzyme level is to eat living, whole foods high in food enzymes which digest themselves in the food-enzyme stomach.

High enzyme content foods are mango, papaya, pineapple, grapes, apple, fresh figs, banana and carob. Cultured foods (foods predigested by the introduction of bacteria) like yogurt and sauerkraut have extra high levels of enzymes. Dried fruits are concentrated in vitamins and minerals which aid enzyme function and are useful during the transition but only as needed since they can damage the teeth.

To increase our level of health we need to increase our bodily levels of enzymes and VITAL LIFE energy (also variously called chi, chee, Qi, Ki) and decrease enzyme-chi loss.

We also need to remove the obstructions to enzyme and life energy movement and circulation by removing excess mucus and toxic material from the body. Life energy is found in food in the form of living, bioactive enzymes, vitamins and minerals. The conservation of the sexual fluids will also retain the chi in the body-mind.

Another factor that is needed is structural soundness of the organs so that the right elimination can be affected by the vital life principle. If the organs have structural damage due to injury or disease, this will impair the ability of the chi to move through the body. Structural damage to the organs also can impede the detoxification process during the transition, causing a slowed result. Some people who's organs have been damaged extensively by disease or by an accident may not be able to be helped. Most people are generally structurally sound and can heal themselves if they go on the transition diet which removes mucus and toxins and increases the flow of chi.

The vital principle heals the body during fasting by removing waste and repairing tissue. The energy used to digest food is used to heal damaged parts of the body, during a complete abstinence from eating. Fasting helps remove obstructions to chi flow and so does eating mucusless foods and following a systematic transition diet.

Why do a long, draining fast which burns up your enzyme reserve at a rapid rate? Why not do a short juice fast and then change your diet for the better and thus cleanse and nourish the body at the same time with enzyme-rich food sources?

You can do a 42 hour fast (dinner to lunch the second day) using juice (fruit juice, vegetable juice) or lemonade (apple juice and lemon juice) or coconut water when ever needed, such as during a cold or sore throat to clean the system.

Skipping breakfast is an 18 hour fast eating at noon. If you keep going drinking liquid until the next morning it will clean up any toxicity that has built up which can cause headache, irritability, stomach-ache, a sore throat, constipation and acne.

Drink as much as three liters per day of juice during your fast, which will stop the hunger pangs and weakness problems during fasting. Break the fast with a raw salad if you are just beginning or fresh fruit if you are more advanced. You will relish the now greatly appreciated food.

HOW LIVING WATER
ENLIVENS YOU

Living water is alive because it contains living enzymes, the spark of life. Enzymes contain the spark of life or 'chi', 'chee', 'ki' as the Chinese call it.

Chi is a form of bioelectric energy uniquely associated with living things. The Chinese have studied this bioelectric "chi" for 5,000 years and discovered that it ran in specific meridians or energy pathways in the body.

This dovetails with the Kirlian photos of the aura (bioelectric field) of living, uncooked foods showing large, bright fields and that of cooked food showing dark small fields.

To be the most vital that you can possible be, eat foods fresh and raw because they have the most "chi" in them. To feel high or euphoric we need to eat foods high in "chi" which is found in living water rich foods.

The fiber doesn't contain the life force or chi only the liquid portion of the fruit or vegetable. This living liquid is "living water". The best source of this living water is naturally grown, fresh fruits. Fruits are 70%-98% living water. Fruits have a much higher content of enzymes by comparison than vegetables.

Aging is associated with the water content of the body. Infants have a water content as high as 77%, an elderly person may have only 45% and an adult has around 60%. The first 10 years of life shows the most dramatic decrease in water content. We are told by health experts to drink 8 glasses of water a day to stay hydrated. On a vegetarian transitional and on a living foods, lacto-vegetarian diet you are being hydrated by the living water in fresh vegetables and fruits and not dead, mineral laden water.

Inorganic minerals in tap and spring water are deposited in the body causing arthritis and artery hardening. Distilled and purified water can drain minerals from the body. The living water found in fruits, vegetables and coconut water is healthier than lifeless; tap (can contain chlorine, arsenic and other toxic chemicals), distilled, filtered, purified, spring or mineral water.

DR. WESTON PRICE SAYS WE DO NOT GET THE COMPLETE VITAMIN D GROUP FROM SUN EXPOSURE

Chapter 16 of Dr. Weston Price's Nutrition and Physical Degeneration states that vitamin D is not found in plants, but must be sought in an animal food, "There is a misapprehension with regard to the possibility that humans may obtain enough of the vitamin D group of activators from our modern plant foods or from sunshine. This is due to the belief viosterol or similar products by other names, derived by exposing ergosterol to ultraviolet light, offer all of the nutritional factors involved in the vitamin D group.

I have emphasized that there are known to be at least eight D factors that have been definitely isolated and twelve that have been reported as partially isolated. Coffin has recently reported relative to the lack of vitamin D in common foods as follows: 1. A representative list of common foods was carefully tested, by approved technique, for their vitamin D content. 2. With the remote possibility of egg yolks, butter, cream, liver and fish it is manifestly impossible to obtain any amount of vitamin D worthy of mention from common foods. 3. Vegetables and fruits do not contain vitamin D.

It will be noted that vitamin D, which the human does not readily synthesize in adequate amounts, must be provided by foods of animal tissues or animal products. As yet I have not found a single group of primitive racial stock which was building and maintaining excellent bodies by living entirely on plant foods."

Vegan diets in the long run are not natural. All cultures known for their longevity have used some animal products. The Sardinian mountain folk, as described in the book *The Blue Zones*, use sheep milk cheese and very little meat, and the Swiss mountain folk, described by Weston Price use cow's milk Swiss cheese. The Hunzas use cheese and yogurt as their primary protein source eating a little meat only on special holidays.

Dr. Michael Holick has been doing research in the vitamin D field for more than 30 years. He happened to be in the right place at the right time as a graduate student at the University of Wisconsin working with one of the authorities in vitamin D, Dr. Hector DeLuca. His PhD project was the actual isolation and identification of the active form of vitamin D, which he did with his roommate and they were also the first to chemically synthesize it.

They gave vitamin D to patients that had bone diseases associated with kidney failure, that were wheelchair bound and they started walking again.

Asked what would be the benefits if we all got enough vitamin D, he responded, "It's almost incalculable, because like I said if you just think about the study that was done in Finland where it can reduce your risk of getting type 1 diabetes by 80%. Studies that have been done in the United States and Europe show it can decrease risk of getting colon cancer and dying of colon cancer by 50%, prostate cancer by 50%, ovarian cancer and breast cancer by almost the same amount. The amount of not only money saved, but the amount of grief and pain and suffering that people go through with these serious chronic diseases, potentially could be avoided."

Dr. Holick treats his patients with 50,000 IU of vitamin D once a week for 8 weeks and then places them on 50,000 IU of vitamin D once every 2 weeks thereafter.

Even if you have enough vitamin D, only 30% of the calcium you eat is absorbed. Ramiel Nagel, who is healing teeth with nutrition, says there are some 1000 vitamin D factors.

ESSENTIAL FATTY ACIDS

The accepted knowledge in nutrition is that there are two polyunsaturated fatty acids (PUFAs) that cannot be made in the body; linoleic acid LA (omega-6 family) and alpha-linolenic acid ALA (omega-3 family). They must be provided by the diet and are known as essential fatty acids. G. O. Burr and his wife M. M. Burr declared that unsaturated fat was essential for rats in 1929 (Burr & Burr) and in 1930 (Burr & Burr) declared that linoleic or omega-6 and possibly other acids were active.

However, subsequent research in 1940 (Schneider, Steenbock & Platz) proved that the Burr and Burr skin syndrome was cured by giving the laboratory rats either "essential fatty acids" or rice bran concentrate. The presumed "essential" unsaturated fat was shown to be unessential because rice bran concentrate containing vitamin B6 and probably combined with a mineral deficiency cured the exact same disease created by the Burr diet.

Burr's basic animal diet was deficient in many different nutrients but in particular vitamin B6. The disease that appeared in Burr's animals could be cured by fat free B-vitamin preparations, or by purified vitamin B6 when it became available, thus proving that there are no "essential fatty acid" deficiency diseases.

In the 1940s, Roger Williams' lab at the Clayton Foundation Biochemical Institute, University of Texas at Austin, recognized the "fat deficiency disease" of the Burrs as a deficiency of vitamin B6, and showed that when they produced the condition with a diet similar to the one the Burrs had used, they could cure it by administering vitamin B6.

Right after the Burr's studies were published in 1929 and 1930 an experiment was done by biochemist W. R. Brown who volunteered to live for six months on a diet extremely low in fat.

He was clinically well throughout the entire period, not having even a common cold. There was a marked absence of fatigue. Attacks of migraine subsided completely. The respiratory quotient rose markedly after a meal. Blood total lipids increased but unsaturation decreased 25%. Linoleic and arachidonic acids decreased about 50%. W. R. Brown did not develop scaly skin or other visible abnormality, fortifying the medical profession's doubt that essential fatty acids had any relevance to humans.

However, this failure to reproduce the disease in a human by depriving him of the essential fatty acids was dismissed giving the excuse that an adult human contained about two pounds of linoleic acid which would require longer than 6 months for depletion.

Dr. Raymond Peat points out that in the 1940s and 1950s most textbooks described the idea that certain fats were essential nutrients, as a controversial idea. He states that, "Although 'Burr's disease' clearly turned out to be a B-vitamin deficiency, probably combined with a mineral deficiency, it continues to be cited as the basis justifying the multibillion dollar industry that has grown up around the 'essential' oils."

The widespread use of seed oils as a fat source only began in the 1940s to 1950s when paints, which formally used seed oils as the base, were being made from petroleum oil. The gigantic seed oil industry didn't want to lose all their profits so they decided to sell their vegetable oils for cooking and salad dressing.

In order to stay in business they used public relations to effectively sell the medical (heart protective) benefits of a diet containing increased amounts of linoleic and linolenic acids as opposed to the now demonized saturated fats, thanks to Ancel Keys in 1953, and basing it all on the 1929 publication by Burr and Burr and ignoring subsequent publications that proved it was a vitamin B6 deficiency.

More recent research has proven that the highly unstable polyunsaturated fats "essential fatty acids" can cause cancer.

A study of cod liver oil (22.5% polyunsaturated fat) intake by over 50,000 Norwegian men and women over a 12-year period found that those taking cod liver oil had three times the risk for melanoma, the most dangerous type of skin cancer (Veierød, Thelle, & Laake, 1997).

Another researcher, ironically named Burr, found that both oily fish and fish oil supplements increased sudden cardiac death. In a study of 3114 men under 70 years of age with coronary heart disease, the first of four groups was advised to eat two servings of oily fish weekly, or to take three capsules of fish oil daily. Another group was advised to eat fruit, vegetables and oats. The third group was given both suggestions, and the fourth group was a control.

In no group was mortality reduced, but in the group that ate oily fish or fish oil capsules, mortality from cardiac death was increased. Those taking the fish oil capsules had an even greater risk of sudden cardiac arrest (Burr et al., 2003). This study shows that even eating oily fish high in polyunsaturated fats (salmon except for chum and pink, tuna, trout, mackerel, herring, sardines) can lead to heart attacks.

Fish oils and especially fish liver oils are often contaminated with mercury, PCBs, pesticides and dioxins. Harsh chemicals like phosphoric acid and then deodorization using steam or molecular distillation removes some of the contaminates, but also renders the fish oil molecules toxic.

A study of 47,000 men has found that ALA omega-3 fatty acids (similar to those found in flax seed oil) may increase the risk of advanced prostate cancer (Leitzmann et al., 2004).

A baby gets fat from human mammalian milk and not processed seeds. Seed oils found in plant seeds were made toxic to humans by Mother Nature, thus helping the survival of the plant species. Unsaturated fats found naturally in mother's milk are fats made for our consumption, whereas seed fat is needed by the seed to reproduce its species.

If you were to give an infant just the essential polyunsaturated fats and no saturated or monounsaturated fats in an infant formula common sense would dictate that the baby would become ill.

Following the logic of the essential fatty acids we only need to consume polyunsaturated fats and not saturated fats or monounsaturated fats since they both are unessential. Naturally occurring saturated fats and unsaturated fats as found in grass-fed dairy products are the real essential fatty acids.

To the infant are not all the fats in mother's milk essential for good health? In 100 grams of human milk 2 grams are saturated fat, 1.7 grams are monosaturated fat and 0.5 grams are polyunsaturated fat.

The human body can convert Omega 3 or alpha-linolenic acid and Omega 6 or linoleic acid to other PUFAs such as arachidonic acid (AA), eicosapentaenoic acid (EPA) and docosahexaenoic acid (DHA) and therefore there is no need to eat fish or take fish oils to get enough DHA or EPA in your diet.

Studies of ALA metabolism in healthy young men indicate that approximately 16% of dietary ALA is converted to long chain omega-3 derivatives; (8% EPA, and 0-4% is converted to DHA) (Burdge et al, 2002).

In healthy young women, 36% of dietary ALA is converted to long chain omega-3 derivatives; (21% EPA, 6% DPA, 9% DHA) (Burdge & Wootton, 2002).

SUPPLEMENTS

"THE FRUIT THEREOF SHALL BE FOR FOOD, AND THE LEAF (HERBS, GRASSES, VEGETABLES) THEREOF FOR HEALING" EZEKIEL 47:12

Lee Ching Yuen lived to be 256 years old as proven by government records in China. His three primary rules of living were never hurry, avoid extreme emotions and observe daily exercise and meditation. He recommended: ginseng, gotu kola, garlic and lycii or goji berries.

Ginseng is the finest herbal tonic. Gotu kola supports the mind and memory and garlic is a super anti-oxidant to help fight toxic free radicals. Use plenty of garlic in salads, tomato sauce and vegetable dishes.

Goji berries are the richest source of carotenoids known, including beta-carotene (having more beta carotene than carrots). They contain 500 times the amount of vitamin C by weight than oranges. The berries contain 18 kinds of amino acids (six times higher than bee pollen) and contain all 8 essential amino acids. Goji berries are imported from Tibet, Mongolia and China and are usually cultivated naturally without chemicals, but it is best to buy certified organic sources. Taking goji berries as a powdered supplement in capsules is an option if you don't want to damage your teeth chewing dried fruit.

Rose hip powder and camu camu are natural sources of vitamin C which helps form collagen in the skin which maintains flexibility and avoids wrinkling. They protect against air, water, chemical and electro-magnetic radiation pollution and other toxins in the environment and prevent plaque formation in the arteries. Rose hip powder can be eaten mashed with berries and banana.

Bee pollen has scientific studies that prove its effectiveness. No less than the United States Department of Agriculture has done research to prove bee pollen's worth. The study titled "Delay in the Appearance of Palpable Mammary Tumors in C3H Mice Following the Ingestion of Pollenized Food," (1948) by William Robinson of the Bureau of Entomology, Agriculture Research Administration. It was published in the Journal of the National Cancer Institute in October, 1948.

Bee pollen research began with the people of the Caucasus Mountains in the former Soviet Union. Doctors began to study them because of their optimum health and longevity. Many of them were healthfully living to over 100 years old. A large percentage of them were beekeepers and it was discovered that the pollen they ate was their magic elixir.

Bee pollen has more amino acids and vitamins than other amino-acid containing products like beef, eggs or cheese. Its nutritional diversity makes bee pollen an ideal dietary supplement and boost to a balanced diet. Scientists have labeled it the most nutritious supplement on the planet.

LIST OF SUPPLEMENTS

1. **Multi-Vitamin:** New Chapter and Megafood are the highest quality food grown vitamins on the market.
2. **Mineral Supplement:** Carob powder (mix with banana and papaya), Alive! Calcium, Flora brand silica, Biosil.
3. **Other Supplements:** The supplements in capital letters listed below are highly recommended, the ones in small case letters can be taken as needed.
A. **Ginseng** Red Korean, American and Siberian. Both women and men can benefit from ginseng. Ginseng nourishes your vital life energy and buffers you from the daily drain of stress. Red Korean ginseng especially supports the sex glands and acts as a natural Viagra.
B. **Bee pollen** A tablespoon a day.
C. **Spirulina** is an excellent protein (55-72%), GLA and mineral source.
D. **Vitamin C** Camu camu powder, rose hip powder, amla powder (Capsules or powder). These are the best natural sources of vitamin C. 1-2 caps or more, if needed, per day.
E. **Senna or Sen** Used when fasting to empty the bowels completely in 4-5 hours. This herb really makes the fast less painful by cleaning out the colon so thoroughly. Use it when you get constipated, bloated and gassy.
f. **Saw palmetto** Male prostate health, 2-3 capsules per day.
g. **Gotu kola** A famous Indian herb to boost mind power.
h. **Nettles tablets** Also Alfalfa and Dandelion, naturally high in calcium and minerals. 2-4 per day.
i. **Goji berries** Nutritionally concentrated.
j. **Plant Enzymes** Plant not animal enzymes, especially bromelain, papain and those from Aspergillus oryzae.
k. **Beta Alanine** 2 to 3 grams per day for a minimum of 4 months. Precursor to making carnosine. To prevent or reverse grey hair, also take copper sebacate 22 mg per day.

l. **Vitamin K2 MK-4** Life Extension's Super K is a good product. Tooth and bone healer. Removes calcium deposits from the arteries.
m. **Vitamin D** Dr. Holick, who first synthesized vitamin D recommends: 50,000 IU of vitamin D-3 or D-2 once a week for 8 weeks and then 50,000 IU of vitamin D once every 2 weeks thereafter.
The following supplements are for people over 50 years of age:
m. **Pregnenolone** 5-10 mg per day, let it dissolve under the tongue to avoid being processed by the liver. Dr. Raymond Peat recommends it as the best thing for wrinkles. He considers it the major anti-aging steroid, good for increasing memory and improving mood. Many aging characteristics such as sagging skin, "chicken neck," bags under the eyes receded when he took it. These changes were dramatically evidenced in a passport photo taken one year before pregnenolone and 10 weeks after pregnenolone therapy was initiated.
n. **Progesterone** Men apply a one inch strip of cream (11 mg progesterone) two times per day to thin skin areas (scrotum, inside arms, wrist, ankles, chest and feet, rotate to improve absorption) according to Dr. John Lee, a leading authority on progesterone. Dr. Lee showed that it reversed prostate cancer in men and reversed osteoporosis in women. Women take 20 mg or a two inch strip applied two times per day. Non-menstruating women take one week off per month. Menstruating women use only from the 14th to the 26th day, counting the day the period starts as the first day.
o. **L-Arginine, Choline, B-5 or Pantothenic Acid** Makes new mitochondria. Also the best vitamins for men to take 45 minutes before having sex are arginine, choline and vitamin B-5. Physicians suggest that a standard dose of L-arginine in pill-form can be one to three grams with a maximum of nine grams in a 24-hour period.
p. **Lipoic acid and Acetyl-L-carnitine** Significantly protected mitochondria from oxidative damage and age-associated decay.
q. **Coenzyme Q-10 (CoQ-10)** Ubiquinol is the reduced form and has far greater water solubility and much better absorption than ubiquinone. Coenzyme Q-10 helps produce ATP, our energy source.
r. **Selenium** Co-factor for the enzyme glutathione peroxidase and aid to thyroid function. For use in prostate cancer prevention take 200 micrograms daily, over 400 micrograms a day in adults, is a toxic overdose.

NUTRIENTS FOR THE PROSTATE AND HAIR

Saw palmetto is an herbal product used in the treatment of symptoms related to prostate swelling. The active component is found in the fruit of the American dwarf palm tree. Many studies have demonstrated the effectiveness of saw palmetto in reducing symptoms associated with benign prostatic hyperplasia (BPH). Saw palmetto appears to have efficacy similar to that of medications like finasteride, but it is better tolerated and less expensive. There are no known drug interactions with saw palmetto and reported side effects are minor and rare.

Saw palmetto blocks DHT (dihydrotestosterone), the hormone that kills hair follicles. Male pattern baldness can be treated successfully thanks to the herb. Saw palmetto is the main ingredient in 90% of all hair loss products although the U.S. National Library of Medicine in Bethesda, Maryland and the National Institutes of Health state that more studies are necessary before saw palmetto can be recommended for this use.

Yet these two prestigious organizations do recommend saw palmetto for prostate health, "numerous human trials report that saw palmetto improves symptoms of benign prostatic hypertrophy (BPH) such as nighttime urination, urinary flow, and overall quality of life, although it may not greatly reduce the size of the prostate.

Although the quality of these studies has been variable, overall they suggest effectiveness. Although a (2003) study by Willetts et al. reported no difference over a 12-week period and a (2006) well-designed study by Bent et al. reported no difference over a 12-month period, overall the weight of available scientific evidence favors the effectiveness of saw palmetto over placebo. Multiple mechanisms of action have been proposed, and saw palmetto appears to possess 5-a-reductase inhibitory activity (thereby preventing the conversion of testosterone to dihydrotestosterone DHT). Hormonal/estrogenic effects have also been reported, as well as direct inhibitory effects on androgen receptors and anti-inflammatory properties."

In a Cochrane Review, conducted by Wilt T. et. al. (2002) a meta-analysis of randomized controlled studies comparing saw palmetto with placebo or other drugs was made. The review combined the results of 21 trials with durations of four to 48 weeks. The 21 studies included a total of 3,139 men with a mean age of 65 years (range: 40 to 88 years). In the 13 studies that reported symptom scores, saw palmetto improved symptom scores, individual symptoms, and flow measures more than placebo. Patients and physicians were more likely to report improvement in symptoms with saw palmetto treatment than with placebo.

Other recent studies that prove saw palmetto is effective for an enlarged prostate are Gerber G. S. et al. (2001), Marks L. S. et al. (2001), Marks L. S., et al. (2000), Small J. K., et al. (1997), Carraro J. C., et al. (1996), Plosker G. L., et al. (1996), Lowe F. C., et al. (1996), Di Silverio F., et al. (1992) and Briley M., et al. (1984). Clinical studies have used a dosage of 160 mg twice daily or 320 mg once daily of a lipophilic extract containing 80 to 90 percent of the volatile oil. A daily dosage of 480 mg was not found to be any more effective in a six month study of dosages. The whole berries can be used at the recommended dosage of 1 to 2 g daily. Saw palmetto is not an expensive supplement, 100 capsules are around $12.00. Saw palmetto is widely used in other countries, for example, it is used in 50 percent of treatments for BPH in Italy and in 90 percent of such treatments in Germany.

Nettle extract has been used to improve hair health by making the hair stronger, thicker and shinier due to its high concentration of vitamins. While no clinical studies have been conducted yet on the use of nettle in treating DHT-related hair loss and male pattern balding, research does indicate that nettle root can prevent the conversion of testosterone to DHT. The good news is that it also helps women to treat hair loss. Nettle oil is probably the most powerful of nettle infusions. Nettle oil should be massaged into the scalp and hair at least once a week.

Brushing the hair 100 times while bending over to enable blood flow to the scalp is an old beauty secret.

Elson M. Haas MD states on page 222 in Staying Healthy With Nutrition (1995), "Acute deficiency (of zinc) may cause hair loss or thinning, dermatitis, and decreased growth. Both poor appetite and digestion are also experienced by adults with zinc deficiency. Loss of taste sensation may occur, as can brittleness of the nails or white spots on the nails, termed leukonykia. These and most other symptoms can be corrected with supplemental zinc. Sulfur may be helpful as well. Skin rashes, dry skin, and delayed healing of skin wounds or ulcers may result from zinc deficiency, and stretch marks, called striae, are also produced by this condition. Zinc and copper are both needed for cross-linking of collagen, and when they are low, the skin tissue may break down."

Tyrosinase is the enzyme needed to maintain hair color. Hydrogen peroxide (H_2O_2) breaks down tyrosinase, the enzyme which enables oxidation of tyrosine into melanin pigment in the hair follicle.

H2O2 also breaks down the enzyme that keeps in check methionine sulfoxide which inhibits the production of tyrosinase. The body makes catalase to break down H2O2 but as we age we produce less.

Carnosine increases catalase production and fights the hydroxyl radicals that attack tyrosinase. The best way to boost catalase and fight the damaging effects of hydrogen peroxide is by taking 2 to 3 grams per day of beta-alanine, a precursor building block to carnosine, for at least 4 months. Copper is essential to tyrosinase function, so in addition take a copper supplement for 4 months. Consuming enough cheese will also make sure you are getting enough amino acids to make carnosine.

Take a multi-vitamin high in zinc, selenium, iodine and magnesium to nourish the thyroid. Tyrosine is needed to make thyroid hormones and to make melanin. Mozzarella cheese has 1249 mg tyrosine in 3.5 oz.

FEED THE SKIN
OIL AND FAT WHICH CONTAIN
THE FAT SOLUBLE VITAMINS A AND E

Fats and oils applied to the skin keep it moisturized and youthful. If you apply oil or fat to the skin the vitamins are absorbed. A daily, morning application of coconut oil, fresh cream, sesame oil, rose hip seed oil, cocoa butter, vitamin E oil etc. during a short 10-15 minute sunbath, is a great emollient for the skin. As we get older we lose some of the natural elasticity and youthful, moisturized condition of the skin. Applying oil will make up for this loss.

WHEATGRASS JUICE

Here are the scientifically proven benefits of wheatgrass juice:

1. Wheat grass is proven to be effective if you have distal ulcerative colitis (Ben-Arye E et al., 2002). The study size was 21 people. This 2002 study tested fresh wheatgrass juice against a sham drink in a group of people with ulcerative colitis. All of them received regular medical care, including their usual diet. Those who drank about 3 ounces of the juice every day for a month had less pain, diarrhea, and

rectal bleeding than those in the group drinking the placebo.

2. Wheat grass is proven to be good for transfusion dependent beta thalassemia, a severe form of anemia. A 25% or more reduction in blood transfusion was realized in 50% of the patients, of which 3 had more than a 40% reduction (Marawaha RK, Bansal D, Kaur S, Trehan A, 2004). The patients consumed about 100 ml (about 3 1/2 ounces) of wheat grass juice daily. 16 people were analyzed.

3. Wheatgrass in conjunction with a living foods (LF) diet has been proven to be effective in reducing risk factors for heart disease and cancer and also benefits patients with rheumatoid arthritis (Hänninen O, Rauma AL, Kaartinen K, Nenonen M, 1999).

The most important study is the one you make with your own body. Try drinking wheatgrass juice, 1 ounce at first, and see how you feel immediately after drinking it on an empty stomach.

Also see how you feel after drinking it everyday for a week. These personal studies are the most important because you can feel and often see the difference immediately.

HUCKSTERS AND CHARLATANS SELLING MAGIC BULLET DRUGS AND SUPPLEMENTS

Both pharmaceutical drug pushers and natural food hucksters are trying to sell us health and longevity by selling magic bullet nutrients or drugs that will miraculously cure all our ills. They both try to convince you that you need their product in order to stay healthy and achieve a long, disease-free life. Charlatans are like those snake oil selling traveling salesmen that existed in the 19th century in the American west. A case in point is fish, cod liver, krill and vegan algae oil to supply DHA, EPA and omega-3 which in excess are known to cause heart disease. Don't fall for their tricks; both from the allopathic drug peddlers and the all natural, magic bullet nutrient salesmen.

A balanced diet based on locally or home grown, chemical free fruits, vegetables and grass-fed cultured milk products is the basis of a sound diet. What we need nutrient-wise should come from our food and drink. Taking a few proven supplements in moderation is good insurance, but chasing the next fad nutrient, super food or drug is just filling the coffers of the money-loving hucksters.

HOW DIET AND STRESS AFFECTS OUR EMOTIONAL WELL-BEING

THE STRESS OF MODERN
LIVING IS KILLING US

Living in concrete cities, breathing exhaust gas and fighting traffic is killing the human race as fast as bad food. Air is the most vital element needed for health, yet mankind breathes car fumes.

Go to the country and the air if measured has 2 to 3 negative ions for every positive one. Go to the city and there's one negative ion to every 300 to 600 positive ions.

The positive ions are air pollutants such as car exhaust, diesel truck exhaust and factory smoke. Negative ions help neutralize excess toxic positive ions.

Living among trees and plants with birds chirping is usually only experienced two weeks a year on vacation. We need to live where we would go on vacation. Man is dying for lack of communion with the natural elements.

Stress kills. According to Dr. Hans Selye, "Every stress leaves an indelible scar, and the organism pays for its survival after a stressful situation by becoming a little older."

Emotions that arise out of threat or deficit - fear, frustration, anger, sadness - have a decidedly toxic feel to them and are associated with the release of specific stress hormones, most notably cortisol.

When someone is under a lot of pressure to meet deadlines or a great change occurs in their normal routine like going back to school or starting a new job with all new people or someone close to them dies or they are being sued, all these things can make a person emotionally stressed.

This constant stress creates a continual flight or fight reaction which causes the body to be always on guard and ready to go. This drains the body of its energy, increases blood pressure and heart rate, increases the breath rate and suppresses the immune system, all of which contribute to disease.

70% of the world's diseases are stress related according to the World Health Organization. Stress is largely caused by struggling against and fighting our environment.

According to Dr. Bruce McEwen Ph.D. daily, low-level stress, a hallmark of modern living, can significantly increase the risk for development of serious disease later in life.

The hormones released by the neuroendocrine system produce subtle injuries to the body's immune system that literally burn us out in our older years.

What is stress? Any state that causes people to lose their equilibrium, whether it be mentally, physically or emotionally.

Mild forms can be beneficial and motivating. Most forms are not beneficial.

Sources of stress are many including environmental; weather, pollens, noise, traffic and pollution.

Social Stressors; deadlines, financial problems, job interviews, presentations, disagreements, demands for time, loss of loved ones.

Physiological; adolescence, menopause in women, illness, aging, injuries, lack of exercise, poor nutrition, inadequate sleep.

Thoughts; when your brain interprets complex changes in your environment and body and determines when to turn on the "emergency response" or the FIGHT OR FLIGHT syndrome.

No two people register stress the same exact way but some indications are: a rise in blood pressure, clenched jaw, tension headaches and shallow breathing.

Advanced cases can force the body to shift into another form of stress management including disrupted sleep patterns, gastrointestinal disturbances (diarrhea, constipation, bloating and cramping), IBS (irritable bowel syndrome or spastic colon).

Chronic stress, can literally ruin the health of a strong, healthy person. Heart disease is a common result.

Mental stress can trigger angina as much as physical stress. Angina is chest pain or discomfort in the shoulders, arms, neck or back that occurs when your heart muscle does not get enough blood. It may also feel like indigestion.

YOUR STATE OF MIND
DEPENDS ON YOUR
STATE OF HEALTH

One's mental sanity is directly related to one's health status, which is especially dependent on one's recent nutritional status.

If one has been eating poorly for instance; meat, potatoes, fried chicken, cereal and milk, hamburgers, French fries and colas as the staples of one's diet, you become nutritionally deficient in enzymes, vitamins and minerals besides congesting your body with mucus and toxic material.

Nutrient deficiency and blood toxemia affects the hormonal, circulatory, digestive and especially the brain-nervous systems causing them to malfunction which leads to all kinds of mental illnesses and disorders.

When one has low blood sugar or overly toxic blood from not eating in a timely manner, one feels insane when the mind goes array with all kinds of angry, violent and hypercritical thoughts.

Dr. George Watson of the University of Southern California and author of *Nutrition and Your Mind* (1972) states: "We have found functional mental illness to be a reflection of a disordered metabolism, principally involving the malfunction of enzyme systems."

He also states, "what one eats, digests, and assimilates provides the energy producing nutrients that the blood stream carries to the brain. Any interference with the nutritional supply lines or with the energy-producing systems of the brain results in impaired functioning, which then may be called poor mental health."

This is why vegetarians and even those who, "eat everything" get emotionally unbalanced. They're not crazy they just have low blood sugar and high blood toxemia causing mental and emotional irritation.

They don't need years of psychotherapy, they just need some good nutritional education.

Low blood sugar and high blood toxemia is that irritating feeling that makes you want to explode in anger or just start crying because your nerves feel like they are being pierced with pins and needles.

The brain uses 25% of the total blood glucose, yet it comprises only 2.5% of the total body weight.

This highly complex and active brain we possess needs a constant source of glucose or else it malfunctions causing emotional imbalance and mental illness.

When you get up in the morning you've been fasting for 10 to 14 hours so you need to slow down the cleansing process and give your body some carbohydrate fuel by having fruit. Filling the stomach stops or slows the elimination. You can bring coconut water, vegetable juice, fruit and even salad in a container, if you are away from home.

If you are experiencing excessive elimination making you feel really poorly, it may be necessary to eat heavier foods in addition to a salad and steamed vegetables like rice, potatoes, rye crisp bread and toasted whole wheat bread. This will slow down your elimination allowing you to feel good emotionally and mentally.

There are three ways glucose is supplied to the brain; glucose rich foods such as grapes which enter the blood directly, the breakdown of carbohydrates (starches or complex carbohydrates) and the breakdown of liver glycogen.

In the traditional Taoist or Chinese medical system;
1. Essence (Jing); hormones, enzymes, semen, ova, vitamins, minerals, glucose provide...
2. Energy (Ching); bioelectric energy to support the...
3. Spirit (Shen); mind.

"Any break in the steady supply of glucose to the brain causes mental impairment the first symptom of which is loss of emotional control.", according to Dr. George Watson.

I have seen this happen many times in myself. I will skip a meal and become weak, irritated and even disturbed mentally to the point where my thoughts and emotions become negative and angry.

Normally you have the strength to control your emotions if someone bumps into you or calls you a name, but when your brain has no blood glucose then you lose your cool much easier and do things that you regret later.

When the blood sugar is low, this is in fact temporary insanity (sane meaning healthy) of the brain.

This also happens when the blood is filled with toxic material from fasting. A short shopping trip can turn into a hellish nightmare if you were hungry when you left!

Many who try fasting and a fruit and vegetable diet get weak and thus blame the food when in reality it's the toxic condition of their bodies and the failure to eat the right foods at the right time.

It's best to avoid skipping meals or eating late when in transition because this upsets the delicate balance between cleansing too fast and cleansing too slowly. Skipping meals speeds up cleansing and eating later at night will slow down cleansing but also can cause indigestion. Going to sleep on a full stomach creates indigestion due to the digestive organs partially shutting down during sleep.

Many diseases are caused by eating heavy foods like meat, eggs and bakery products which clog the body with mucus and toxins but another disease is caused by eating too lightly, skipping meals, fasting, eating only fruit or only raw food, all of which will over-stress the body causing mental imbalance.

Anorexia really becomes dangerous when the person becomes extremely weak and thin, yet stubbornly believes they are on the right path.

PESTICIDES CAN AFFECT
THE NERVOUS SYSTEM

Another cause of emotional imbalance is eating agro-chemically treated fruits and vegetables. Pesticide contaminated food can give you the jitters or make you nervous. Many pesticides were created during W.W. II to be used for chemical warfare.

They are potent, nervous system affecting chemicals that can cause numbness, headache, nervousness, paralysis, cancer and even death. People have been paralyzed for life by parathion, the organophosphate pesticide, which is still used in the United States, although banned in many countries around the world.

This is an extremely important point; this diet only works with organically grown or naturally grown (without chemicals) fruits and vegetables.

If you can't afford certified organically grown produce, then seek out farmer's markets where the farmers use natural methods or are so poor they can't afford pesticides.

You also can experiment with produce by eating it, then waiting to see if you get a headache or numbness or a light headed feeling, which indicates it was sprayed with pesticides.

TOWARDS AN ENLIGHTENED PSYCHOLOGY

Mankind is generally caught in feelings of inadequacy, dissatisfaction, alienation, desperation and confusion.

He/she is afflicted with the "two diseases", or the belief in a permanent, spatially separate personality or self based on the material senses (the inner disease) and the belief in the reality of external objects based on impermanent matter (the outer disease), with the hope that they can provide ultimate satisfaction. "I can't get no, satisfaction.", sang the Rolling Stones. The illusory, separate, material sense-based self-conception will never find satisfaction, only by identifying with your Immortal Spirit, the Ideal, Divine Man/Woman can you find true contentment and permanent satisfaction. The ego or sense-based self is made up of body, feelings, perceptions, mental thoughts based on the senses, and consciousness. All of these components of the personality are impermanent and constantly changing. The external material world is likewise constantly changing. Exposing the falsity of the spatially separate, ego self and personality and understanding the transitory, unlasting nature of all external objects frees one from the two great diseases. How to do this is to understand the illusion of the two diseases and then start living a more spiritual, simplified life. We can become too complicated by the world and all its illusory distractions. The simple life living in the country or suburbs growing fruits and vegetables, reading and writing books, taking walks in nature, making artistic creations like books, songs, paintings, crafts, clothes, tools, beautiful gardens, is the way to remain reflective and contemplative of the ground of our being.

It's like saying, "Yes, the world is a beautiful, terrible, radiant manifestation, yet it's still a radiance or a motion picture, an illusion that we must see through to the Divine, Who will embrace us as His own in mutual recognition." We need to see that we are really, in essence, the Son of Man, the Ideal Adam/Eve, the Eternal Human, Who never fades away, but at the same time revering all creation as being infused with Divinity. It maybe impermanent, but we still need to love and respect creation.

Humans were made from matter and breathed to life by God's Spirit, yet our true, ideal form is spiritual not material. If we follow the true, inner Spirit and not a counterfeit substitute we will return to the ideal.

We must avoid falling into the trap of thinking that the spiritual exists apart from us and only in Heaven, the Eternal Paradise. We are Eternal Spiritual Souls and the Divine Eternal Realm is our true spiritual home, yet we live on the temporal earth with all its distractions and impermanence. We can be free from this lesser, impermanent, material world if we trust in the Eternal Spirit. This idea could make us loathe or hate this world, when really we need compassion and wisdom to love the material world and all its limitations.

We can love the earth by living in a material, albeit transient paradise garden and then prepare ourselves for the Eternal Spiritual Realm. We can spiritualize our body and mind through right diet, knowledge and action. We can enliven our physical bodies with Spirit. A living water diet (bread of life translated correctly in the bible) allows us to be born again in Spirit. This was the real Baptism of John.

Paradise really is an intuited awareness of the Eternal Spirit within us in each moment and therefore is not dependent on the physical location. That being said it is easier to intuit the Divine in a natural, peaceful, country location than in a noisy, polluted city.

CONSERVATION OF SEXUAL VITALITY

The benefits people accrue from the conservation of semen and the reduction or elimination of menstruation are increased vitality, strength, endurance, creativity, drive, zestfulness, emotional well being, freedom from back, joint and leg pain, a sparkle in the eyes and color in the face, less wrinkles in the complexion and a more sensitive, caring demeanor. The semen is the most vital and precious substance that a man has. It's his elixir of life and the fountain of youth if it's conserved and nourished by vital, enzyme-rich, living foods.

The semen can be controlled by the mind and the contraction of the anal sphincter muscles. By avoiding excess stimulation, the point of no return, where one cannot prevent ejaculation, is avoided. A full bladder can put pressure on the seminal vesicles creating a desire to ejaculate when really all you need to do is urinate.

A man can have an orgasm or multiple orgasms without the loss of semen, wherein the prostate gland contracts just like in an ejaculatory orgasm with the same pleasurable feeling. This can be learned through masturbation wherein the semen is retained and the feeling of orgasm is experienced through the contraction of the prostate gland rather than the loss of semen.

One can stimulate oneself in masturbation and learn to contract certain muscles so the semen is retained but the orgasm is felt as a thrilling, earth moving, ecstatic feeling. If the semen wants to ejaculate, one can draw it up by contracting the anal sphincter muscles firmly and by also exhaling all one's air, then pulling in the abdomen like is done in yogic exercises. More often than not, urine in the bladder creates the desire to ejaculate semen. After urinating one will have the control to reach an orgasm, without the loss of semen.

Taoists emit semen in the spring but less and less as they get older. Young men can get away with it, but not older men. There are too many hormones, which an older man is not producing like he did in his youth, for him to waste his semen. Avoiding ejaculation can be trained into the mind over time through practice and trial and error. Always protect yourself and your partner if you have not mastered control of the semen by using contraceptives to avoid pregnancy.

Karezza means caress in Italian and is pronounced Ka-ret-za. Karezza is the art of making love without the goal being orgasm. It's slow love, making love the long way, not short and passionate. It's about uniting two beings in oneness physically, mentally and spiritually. A good position to avoid excess stimulation, is where the women straddles or gets on top of the man in the seated or lying position. The man can sit on a pillow for more support and comfort. At first remain motionless and feel the energy in the genitals. The seated position will give less stimulation than the lying position, so it's best to start with this position. There is a pleasant energy that radiates from the man's perineum (between the anus and scrotum, base chakra) into the woman's vagina, up toward her breasts, then out from her to your chest, down your body back toward your genitals, then out into her again.

The man should open his heart and cultivate loving feelings and kindness to the woman. The male gives his positive energy through the penis and it is taken in by the female who transforms it and sends it back to the man through her breasts. Allow the penis to slowly expand and grow inside of the woman.Focus on relaxing and away from getting swept away by the temptation of moving quickly and getting heated up. It's best to remain perfectly still. Stay with it and wait, you will learn that there is an incredible gift for both of you which is a deep, feeling of peace, light and spiritual serenity. In time with patience and practice you can experience a supernatural feeling of oneness and rejuvenation wherein you feel stronger and younger after lovemaking instead of tired and sleepy.

The position with the female straddled on top of the male is called yab-yum (meaning father-mother) in the Tibetan tradition. This is the non-dual or not two but one position. Eve came out of Adam and they are thus one. Gnostics are dualistic in the sense that their is knowledge (gnosis) of good and evil or the eternal and the transient. Gnostics are non-dualistic in the sense that Humans are one with Spirit, albeit less than the Trinity of God the Father, Barbelo His Emanation and Christ Their Son. In Platonic Love (Eros) is the desire to possess the good (or true beauty) forever. This desire is not only the openly sexual kind, but also the businessman's and worker's desire of riches, the artist's desire of beautiful works, or the philosopher's love of wisdom. All lovers desire to create, either children, or more intellectual things such as art works and political systems. By being creative lovers they achieve some sort of immortality. The beauty and offspring of the mind are more honorable than those of the body or having children and also material wealth, objects of art, buildings and gardens. The most admirable lovers are those who move from the love of the physical and individual to the love of the intellect/virtue/character and general. This is the true meaning of Platonic love. It is non-physical love and pro-virtue/character/intellect (brightness, light) love. If a relationship was based on spiritual beauty and not physical beauty then it could include physical love as a secondary consumation but not for the purpose of procreation ideally rather for co-recreation or the healing power of sexual energy.

NATURAL LIVING,
ITS ORIGIN AND RELATION
TO OUR HEALTH

HEALTH TO HUMANS,
BALANCE TO THE EARTH

Why is there so much disease and suffering in the world? What went wrong? Or do we even care anymore being resigned to how things are? Something is definitely wrong, just look at the environmental destruction, the proliferation of disease and the escalation of wars and terrorism.

Are we here to become as rich and famous as possible and live in exorbitant luxury or is there another road less taken that we have somehow lost along the way? Is there a way of living that will make us healthy and happy and also be healthy for the earth, because obviously something is wrong with what we are doing now.

Look at all the devastation that is going on in the world ecologically, what with the rainforests being cut down, the climate crisis and the loss of prime agricultural soil and it's all getting worse as the population increases every year!

Could we create paradise on earth? An ecological garden that provides our food and normalizes the climate? Could each person or family start producing most of their food in their own paradise garden? Could we live a simple, natural life with all the basic, modern conveniences as part of it, yet powered by non-polluting renewable energy like solar and wind power?

The most densely populated area in India is Kerala and in it are some 3.5 million forest gardens. These sustainable farming systems generate astounding yields; a plot of just 0.12 hectare or 1/3 of an acre can contain 23 coconut palms, 12 clove trees, 56 banana plants, 49 pineapple plants and 30 pepper vines trained up the trees. A model of efficient and sustainable agriculture, Kerala produces more than any other Indian state agriculturally and its population is 100% literate. On the Physical Quality of Life Index Kerala rates higher than any other Asian country except Japan, despite being one of the most densely populated places on earth.

Kerala is located in a tropical environment which makes it easier in winter but a sub-tropical climate is about the same. Temperate climates need more adaptation during the winter. Greenhouses help to extend the growing season. Temperate food storage of apples, root vegetables and cabbages provides a food supply in the dormant winter season.

Multiplying these mini-gardens all over the earth would create a balanced ecological system. The tree's evaporation and shade moderates hot, dry climates, holds water in its roots preventing topsoil erosion and fertilizes the soil from fallen leaves and branches.

Forest or orchard gardening is an ancient way of truly civilized living that creates health in our bodies and ecological balance on the earth. The wealth of nations is their health both physical and environmental. If we feed the body properly and live a natural life, the mind thinks good thoughts, the emotions are elated and the spirit communes with God in an ecologically balanced, paradise garden.

The choice is ours, we can live in balance, which means conservation of existing forests, reforestation and sustainable, forest fruit gardens, or imbalance which means further deforestation of our tropical and evergreen forests and expansion of industrialized factory farms resulting in pollution, disease and climate destabilization.

PARADISE:
WHERE NATURAL LIVING BEGAN

"Folk tales are haunted with remembrance of an ancient day when men lived in a Paradise Garden abounding with juicy sweet fruit. With the Hebrews it was the Garden of Eden, with the Celts, the lost island of Avalon; with the Greeks, that wonderful garden on an island in the Western seas the Hesperides; with the Persians, the Haoma-Tree Paradise; with the Chinese, the garden of the Peach Tree Goddess...", writes Henry Bailey Stevens (1949).

The image of paradise rings throughout cultural history: the Elysian fields of the Greeks, Plato's Republic, Ovid's Golden Age, Valhalla of the Norse gods, the Inca's city of gold, Cortez's El Dorado, the Australian Aborigine's Dream Age, Dante's Paradise, Thomas More's Utopia, the Wizard of Oz's Emerald City, Atlantis, Hilton's Shangri-La and Buddhism's Shambhala.

The word paradise brings many things to mind; a garden of trees and grassy meadows, birds chirping, the sound of a gurgling creek, colorful fruits laid out on tablecloths on the grass, people laughing and playing like it's Sunday afternoon.

The story of paradise is where we get our idea of a life close to nature, of a man and a woman living simply in a peaceful garden. It motivates us to make money and retire early to live in a warm, sunny place. We search for lovers and marry to reclaim the integral bliss we felt when we were one with God in the Garden. Paradise or oneness with the eternal, Divine Mind, is the happiness we all so fervently pursue because it's indelibly imprinted in the memory of our DNA.

In An Encyclopedia of Archetypal Symbolism (1991) we learn the English word paradise derives from the Old Persian pairidaeza, which means a walled enclosure, pleasure park or garden. The word pairidaeza entered Hebrew, Aramaic and Greek while still retaining its original meanings.

Paradise is an archetypal image deeply embraced in our collective human unconscious. Was it just a mythical legend or did it really exist?

What does the cultural and scientific evidence show us? What was their diet and what was their lifestyle? These are the questions we will explore in this book.

"In the First Age there was but one religion, and all men were saintly...There were no gods...and there were no demons. The First Age was without disease; there was no lessening with the years; there was no hatred, or vanity, or evil thought whatsoever; no sorrow, no fear. In those times, men lived as long as they chose to live and were without any fear of death.", from the Mahabharata, the spiritual epic of India.

The term "golden age", a time of greatness, originated from early Greek and Roman poets who remembered an ancient time when man was pure and the world a paradise.

The Garden of Eden in the Old Testament is derived from Sumerian and Akkadian myths. Sumeria is considered by many the oldest known civilization in the world (approximately 3000 B.C) having developed the first handwriting system.

The Sumerian paradise is called Dilmun. Eden or edinu was also originally a Sumerian word, meaning a plain or steppe. Dilmun was an earthly garden where sickness and death did not exist.

The creation story where the world is created in seven days is derived from the Babylonian myth called Enuma Elish which was unearthed in the nineteenth century by British archaeologists.

The Hebrews were taken in exile to Babylonia (a product of the union of the Akkadians and the Sumerians) in 587 B.C. and thus absorbed these epic myths into their own Genesis in the Old Testament.

Fruit trees in the area of Malaya-Sumatra-Java are the result of long selection and cultivation. Breadfruit, bananas and pineapple, so widely found over the eastern world, do not seed themselves naturally but have to be planted in order to grow. Thus, Dr. Oakes Ames, research professor at Harvard estimated that man must have practiced plant breeding for about 500,000 years.

The hand axe used to cut trees, roots, etc. and to plant much like we use a mattock, was estimated to have existed 500,000 years ago, to match the age of man, but now scientists are already up-dating mankind's age into millions of years from oldest fossil remains. This shows tree and plant culture tools have been made for millions of years, while the spears, arrows, etc. of hunters may go back much less.

"All the available evidence," says Elliot Smith, "seems to point clearly to the conclusion that until the invention of the methods of agriculture and irrigation on the large scale practiced in Egypt and Babylon, the world really enjoyed some such Golden Age as Hesiod described. Man was not driven into warfare by the instinct of pugnacity but by the greed for wealth and power which the development of civilization was itself responsible for creating."

THE ORIGINAL LIFE-STYLE OF HUMANS

When you look at and smell beautiful fruits doesn't it send you to another plane of primordial beauty? When you walk into a beautiful fruit and flower garden or a lush green forest with a creek flowing through it, doesn't it send you to a place beyond time? That's our genetic memory recalling paradise.

Eating fresh fruits and caring for a garden paradise is what the paradise life is all about. Paradise lies within in a balanced body-mind and without in a proverbial Garden of Eden.

Paradise is our natural state, our ground of being, our original home on earth. This simple way of life has the power to transform your life and the lives of everyone on the planet.

Ecological destruction can be traced back to the "fall" from paradise and the eventual cutting of the garden trees to grow grains for bread and raise cattle for meat.

The health crisis in heart disease and cancer and the ecological climate crisis can be traced back to changing our diet from fresh fruits and vegetables to meat, cooked bread and the cutting of the original paradise forest garden.

The simple plan for saving our health and our planet is to plant a fruit and vegetable garden paradise and live off the produce it provides. This gets us back to our roots, to our original, natural diet and way of life.

St. Francis was asked what he would do if he were told he would die that evening, and he replied he would continue working in the garden just like he's doing because that's exactly what he wanted to be doing more than anything else on earth.

Gardening is the noblest vocation. By planting fruit bearing trees we are helping to restore the world-wide balance of carbon dioxide in the air, which is in excess right now creating the greenhouse gas effect, which is warming global temperatures creating climate extremes.

By fertilizing trees with ground rock powder we are restoring the mineral balance of the soil, which has been depleted by the growing of grains and by the natural growth of forests during the last ten thousand years.

Human activity can alter the global climate due to the large scale impact on the environment from forest cutting and carbon dioxide, methane and other greenhouse gas emissions from power plants, vehicles and livestock.

Non-human solar activity such as sunspots and solar flares also have an impact on global warming and cooling. The climate is in a crisis on a world-wide scale due to man-made and natural causes and we can lessen the human impact by conservation and by living a simpler, more natural lifestyle.

Living on living foods one becomes lighter and more buoyant as though you were being lifted up. Living water rich foods wash the body clean with spiritual energy and vivaciousness.

Eat life to feel more alive and in tune with the Inner Living God. Eat living food and one begins to commune with the eternal Spirit and know the Wisdom of God naturally. One feels connected and at peace with themselves because they are in tune with their own inner Spirit.

Meditating for hours daily can't make up for the errors one makes in the selection of one's daily food. Every meal creates a biochemical state of balance and harmony or imbalance and disharmony.

On the cellular level the eating of junk foods high in refined sugar, flour and salt creates a biochemical imbalance which destroys the harmony of the body and mind.

People on omnivorous diets of cooked foods, meat, eggs, bread and a small amount of fruits and vegetables become acidic which makes them feel bad and so they crave cigarettes, coffee and alcohol to alkalize their acidity and thereby make them feel good.

When you transition gradually to a diet high in fresh fruits and vegetables, refined, devitalized food will be rejected as poisons by your now naturally euphoric and highly sensitized body-mind.

LIVING IN NATURE IS
ANOTHER KEY
TO A HEALTHY LIFE

Right actions or one's daily lifestyle creates a happy and healthy life. Right action is freedom from suffering. Wrong action is slavery to suffering.

The lawful order of the universe rewards right actions with pleasure and happiness and wrong actions with pain and misery.

We are our habits. By living an enlightened lifestyle, one becomes enlightenment or happiness itself. Besides food there's one's environment affecting the amount of pleasure and happiness in your life.

Have you ever gone camping in the high mountains and felt charged with energy? That's the effect of prana or chi or life energy in the air which is very concentrated in the mountains, beaches and deserts.

Food is important, but so is a life close to nature. Either living on a farm in the mountains or having a backyard paradise garden, one needs the physical contact with the earth, the air, the sun, the water and the trees. These are the sacred, natural elements for us to commune with.

Working in a garden, caring for the trees and plants, is a healthy profession. It's what we were naturally designed to do.

SUNBATHING IS AN ESSENTIAL PART
OF NATURAL LIVING

"The Way of Natural Living" includes sunbathing, air bathing, water bathing, exercising, fruit cultivation, organic gardening, meditating, contemplating, studying the world's wisdom teachings and writing and teaching in order to share your experience and revelations.

Sunbathing in a bathing suit, underwear or in the nude is another source of food. Just 5 to 10 minutes on each side is all that's needed to get your supply of ultraviolet nourishment.

Light skinned people will need less exposure time. Light entering the eyes stimulates the endocrine glands preventing those stuck-in-the-house-all-day blues.

Short exposure time prevents skin cancer as does a natural diet free of toxic agro-chemicals and rich in antioxidants. Some native people like the aborigines of Australia are in the sun all day but don't have problems with skin cancer.

There is a correlation between skin cancer and excess sun exposure in a toxic, unhealthy body. Polyunsaturated fats as found in commercial cooking oil can cause skin cancer. A Norwegian study found that those taking cod liver oil (very high in polyunsaturated fat) had three times the risk for melanoma, the most dangerous type of skin cancer (Veierød, Thelle, & Laake, 1997).

The body will excrete toxic material while sweating in the sun which in contact with your skin can create an irritation which can lead to the formation of skin cancer by the body as a reaction to these chemicals.

The morning and early afternoon sun from 8 to 2 pm has been shown to be the most beneficial for sunning. The early morning sun is probably the most beneficial and also it's not as hot at these hours creating a more pleasurable experience.

Taking a daily sunbath whenever possible puts a healthy color on your cheeks and a glow in your skin. A little olive or sesame oil or even fresh cow's cream applied to the skin magnifies the sun's rays and also moisturizes the skin.

The skin absorbs nutrients like vitamin E and A contained in the oil just like it can absorb pesticides. Vitamin D, which aids in calcium absorption, is manufactured by sunlight hitting the skin. Who knows what other undiscovered beneficial processes occur taking a sun bath.

Overly tanned people have wrinkled old skin. Old skiers and surfers who didn't use a sun block look old and ragged. The sun can damage the skin if you expose yourself too much.

Moderate exposure is the key to looking sun-kissed and healthy. The sun makes the skin look bronze and beautiful. A tanning salon or skin bronzers are just not as healthy as living in the tropics or sub-tropics where the sun shines just about all year round.

Sunglasses screen out the beneficial rays which help the endocrine glands function, so it's best to only use them when there is excessive glare.

THE HEALING
POWER OF EXERCISE

EXERCISE

Children and young people are very active physically, participating in school sports, gym, recess and after school game playing. This keeps their bodies firm and shapely. Older people, who are no longer in high school or college need to remain physically active to maintain their form. They need a work-out program to stay in shape.

Gardening is a very natural form of exercise, then there is walking, running, weight training, yoga, stretching, basketball, tennis, football, baseball and soccer all of which help keep the body in good firm muscle tone.

If you do farm labor, landscaping or housecleaning for a living then you might think you don't need to exercise. I think this is a mistake because you still need to tone your muscles with weights and move your body to stay healthy. Intentional, concentrated work-outs keep you in the best shape.

The idea of physical culture is not to bolster the ego by having the best physique, rather it's to maintain good physical fitness which helps the mind stay disciplined. If you look and feel good you tend to do good. Discipline of the body helps the mind to stay disciplined and not to wander off in extravagant desires of sensual pleasure, money accumulation and worldly fame.

The first exercise we were given was working in the garden. Digging and heavy pruning can be hard physical work equivalent to doing heavy weight lifting or running sprints. Then there is the lighter gardening movements like light weeding, planting and harvesting.

Gardening is good exercise because you are outside in the fresh air and in contact with the soil. Gardening is good but to keep all your muscles in shape additional exercises are needed such as walking, running and weight lifting.

Weight training is the best way to keep your muscles young and shapely looking. This is because weight lifting isolates and develops specific muscles.

A good way to start off an exercise session is to walk a few minutes and then do some uphill sprints without getting to the heavy panting, out of breath stage. This will warm you up for weight lifting. Sprinting up a hill is an intense cardio and leg/buttocks work-out. You could also use a bicycle or a stationary bicycle or go swimming or play basketball or whatever you enjoy doing.

A few light yoga postures are good to stretch out tight muscles which in turn helps you relax. You can do yoga stretching on the days you are not working out. Remember never to force your muscles to stretch or you could cause back problems. Start by opening wide your legs while sitting on the ground then touch your right hand to your left foot and vice versa. Then lean forward with arms straight and touch the ground in front of you, but never forcing it. Then put your left foot on the inner thigh of your right leg and touch your calf or toes. Feel the stretch. Next put your left foot on the other side of your right thigh and put your right forearm across your left leg so it touches the ground on the other side. Turn your upper body to the left and look behind you feeling the stretch. Never strain. Do the other leg the same. Then roll over on your stomach with your cheek resting on the ground. Lift your head up without using your arms at first and then use your arms to arch up even higher. Come back down and rest deeply by exhaling. Next grab your right foot with your right hand and your left foot with your left hand. Pull on your legs and arch up slowly feeling the stretch in your thighs. Hold the arched position for a moment then slowly lower down. Next raise up your head without using your hands and your feet at the same time as high as possible without straining. Lower slowly then exhale and relax completely.

After the cardio, lift weights with the muscles warm and stretched. A 110 lbs weight set can often be found for around $50.00 USD. This lighter weight set is good for people over 45 and for women. For the younger men needing more weight you may want to invest in a 300 lb. Olympic weight set with a bench, incline bench, decline bench and a rack or you could join a gym. One needs to use as much weight as possible to create muscle mass and size, but not too much weight which can risk injuring your lower back, knees, wrists or ankles. Weight lifting helps keep the muscles toned and large as one eats lighter, water-rich vegetables and fruits.

Warming up with light weights and increasing the weight until one can only do 6 to 3 repetitions (reps), really increases muscle size and density. High reps with light weight will keep the body too lean and skinny.

Weights can be lifted in the evening before retiring if it's too hot during the day or it's too cold in the morning. Always focus on your weakest body part. My weakest body parts are my triceps, shoulders, gluts (the buttock), thighs and calves. My bicep, chest and back are genetically well-muscled.

The physical fitness guidelines (2007) of the American Heart Association (AHA) and the American College of Sports Medicine (ACSM) for healthy adults under age 65 are the following:

Do moderately intense cardio 30 minutes a day, five days a week. Or

Do vigorously intense cardio 20 minutes a day, 3 days a week And Do eight to 10 strength-training exercises, eight to 12 repetitions of each exercise twice a week.

Moderate-intensity physical activity (walking is the best example) means working hard enough to raise your heart rate and break a sweat, yet still being able to carry on a conversation. The 30-minute recommendation is for the average healthy adult to maintain health and reduce the risk for chronic disease.

For adults over age 65 (or adults 50-64 with chronic conditions, such as arthritis) the Guidelines are: Do moderately intense aerobic exercise 30 minutes a day, five days a week.

Or Do vigorously intense aerobic exercise 20 minutes a day, 3 days a week. And Do eight to 10 strength-training exercises, 10-15 repetitions (2-3 more repetitions) of each exercise twice to three times per week.

If you are at risk of falling, perform balance exercises. Have a physical activity plan.

Both cardio and muscle-strengthening activity is critical for healthy aging. Moderate-intensity cardio exercise means working hard at about a level-six intensity on a scale of 10. You should still be able to carry on a conversation during exercise.

Older adults or adults with chronic conditions should develop an activity plan with a health professional to manage risks and take therapeutic needs into account. This will maximize the benefits of physical activity and ensure your safety.

Older adults (over 65 or those 50-64 with chronic conditions like arthritis) do a few more repetitions on the weights and also it is recommended they do it two or three times per week.

So, you are basically working out with weights two or three times a week, in which time you can do cardio as a warm-up for the weights. If you lift weights just twice a week then on another day go running, fast walking, biking, walking up and down hills, swimming or play sports for a minimum of 20 vigorous and intense minutes.

The above is the recommended official exercise plan. Doing five days of cardio instead of weights I would not recommend because strength training is what keeps you looking good. Cardio exercises work the calf and thighs but what about the shoulders, chest, arms and stomach.

It should be noted that if you are overweight or obese, to lose weight or maintain weight loss, 60 to 90 minutes of physical activity may be necessary.

Long, slow cardio (long walks or runs or bike rides) simply doesn't work because it doesn't work both processes of your heart; it doesn't work all three muscle fiber types, nor your three energy systems. The research is so clear about the superior benefits of this type of exercise that the American Heart Association and the American College of Sports Medicine have now totally changed their exercise cardio guidelines, according to Phil Campbell developer of the Peak-8 training workout.

The body does not produce human growth hormone (HGH) after long, slow exercise. Only the short, quick burst anaerobic type of exercise, for short periods of time accomplish this. When you work the fast twitch fiber and work your heart muscle anaerobically, your body releases as much as a 530 percent increase over baseline levels in growth hormone exercise-induced growth hormones (HGH) (Stokes, Nevill, Hall, & Lakomy, 2002). This mimics taking injections of growth hormones.

The (HGH) stays in your body for two hours after the workout burning fat as you rest. There is no HGH test for Olympic athletes anymore because Peak 8 type exercise can mimic taking growth hormones.

The importance of recovery cannot be overstated. How to know if you are recovered from your exercise is when you have a restless energy and you feel like you really want to work out. Sometimes you feel guilty about not working out even if you are tired, but that's the worst time to work out.

Once you are doing intense peak exertion exercises you only need to work out once a week in order to maximize your HGH production.

If you work-out when tired you will just produce the stress hormone cortisol. The Peak 8 protocol takes just 20 minutes once per week because it's that intense and you should not overdo it. You can lift weights afterwards also doing intense slow movements with no rest between sets.

This is all well and good, however there is a another point of view concerning human growth hormone (HGH).

Dr. Raymond Peat, with a PhD in biology and a specialization in physiology says that human growth hormone is a stress hormone and therefore we should avoid the production of this hormone.

He points out that HGH is very high during heart failure, and edema or water retention in the muscles contributes to this problem. HGH causes edema and the increased muscle weight following GH (growth hormone) treatments is due to edema, not "growth."

Heat or hot weather (but not cold weather), hypoglycemia, running and some kinds of shock are known to stimulate HGH production sometimes to levels 10 or 20 times higher than normal. HGH increases during sleep as do the other stress hormones; adrenalin, cortisol and prolactin whereas the beneficial thyroid hormone and progesterone hormone decrease at night.

Estrogen induces a pro-aging, free radical, nitric oxide which releases HGH. All three produce edema (increased fluid retention). Estrogen causes increased secretion of HGH. HGH treatments have produced carpal tunnel syndrome, myalgia, tumor growth, gynecomastia (enlarged breasts in men) and many other problems.

So, there you have it, human growth hormone or HGH is a hormone that you want to avoid producing. Anaerobic exercise or exercise that makes you gasp and breathe hard stimulates the production of HGH to compensate for the stress. So, if you do sprints uphill or use an aerobic gym machine just exercise until you still feel strong but not out of breath. Don't overstress your body which causes it to release HGH.

Yoga is a good exercise because you are not getting out of breath. Weight lifting should be done with heavy weights but don't strain so you get out of breath.

Aerobic exercise is really anaerobic exercise. Getting out of breath means that you no longer are using oxygen to create energy but now are using a non-oxygen way of burning fuel called an- (or without) -aerobic (with oxygen) energy production. Aerobic exercise was made famous by a book published in 1968, but it has been proven wrong.

T3 or thyroid hormone production is stopped very quickly by even "sub-aerobic" or sub-winded exercise. Strenuous exercise is stressful exercise and unhealthy. In a healthy person, rest will tend to restore the normal level of T3, but there is evidence that even very good athletes remain in a hypothyroid state even at rest.

So, what is healthy exercise? The answer is exercise that you can do while still being able to hold a conversation. Swift walking, short sprints uphill, lifting heavy weights with low repetitions, sit-ups, pull-ups, push-ups, yoga and gardening all can be done without stress or without getting out of breath.

The "slender muscles" of long distance runners are signs of a catabolic state, that has been demonstrated even in the heart muscle. A chronic increase of lactic acid and cortisol indicates that something is wrong.

Distance running elevates adrenaline which causes increased clumping of platelets and accelerated blood clotting. Hypothyroidism slows the heart rate and raises the production of adrenalin, and is strongly associated with heart disease.

A slow heart beat means there is a hypothyroid condition. Hypothyroidic people (cold hands and feet) are likely to produce lactic acid even at rest and are especially susceptible to the harmful effects of "aerobic" exercise.

Anaerobic exercise (getting out of breath) increases the release of lactic acid and interleukin-6 from the exercised muscle itself and hormones including estrogen, prolactin, HGH and sometimes TSH (thyroid stimulating hormone) all of which are stress reactions. These substances try to repair the damage done by the stressful exercise, but the price to pay is that the body gets a little older and weaker.

Professional athletes are generally considered to have "good genes," and exercise is said to promote good health, however world class athletes, including participants in the Olympics, have a high incidence of asthma which is about three times higher than the general population.

Exercise physiologists found that "concentric" contraction (when a muscle contracts against resistance like in weight lifting or running up a hill), improves the muscle's function and causes no injury. Running down a hill or eccentric exercise injures the muscles, by forcing them to elongate while bearing a load.

Old people, with very damaged mitochondrial DNA, were given a program of concentric exercise. Over time as they adapted to the program their mitochondrial DNA was found to have become normal. Concentric exercise like weight lifting and short, non-winded, uphill sprints make you physiologically younger.

Short sprints uphill or walking fast uphill is a good warm-up for weight lifting. Don't overdo it on sprinting or walking. Go as fast and as long as is comfortable. A nice walk in the park or woods is much more pleasant and burns more calories (because your brain is taking in the scenery), than using a treadmill machine in a gym. You can walk on the flat parts and sprint up the hills to make it work your legs and calves more. If you are breathing too hard that means you are stressing your body.

LEGS

Shaping the legs and buttocks is easy with the following exercises. Warm up with 5-10 minutes of non-stressful cardio; walking, running, biking or swimming.

A well equipped gym is nice but I work out at home. When doing squats I put on two pairs of pants or one pair of snug fitting jeans to simulate using knee wraps. A tight fitting pair of just washed and dried jeans give your knees and back extra support.

Place the bar behind your neck and shoulders and then squat down until the top of your thigh is parallel to the floor then come up without bouncing. If you work out in a gym the Cybex squat rack will guide your movement. Put a bench under you so you don't go down too low, which can damage your knees, but don't sit on the bench, which can damage your back from all the weight being thrust on your spinal column.

Warm-up with a lighter weight. Then add enough weight to do 3-6 repetitions. Higher reps build endurance but don't build muscle mass. 3-6 reps will build muscle mass. I do one set of back squats, then without rest do front squats and then rest and do another set. This is really 4 sets of squats. Then I do 2 sets of hack squats using a heavy weight to just eek out 6 repetitions. These weight sets done once a week will make your legs well built without much stress and time.

Thigh Exercises

Hack Squats: Hack squats are my favorite exercise to work the thighs. Place a barbell behind you on the ground and then squat down and grab it with both hands and lift up the bar behind your legs. Use a lighter weight to warm-up for one or two sets and then use as much weight as you can to do 3-6 repetitions. Using heavy weight and then going for the burn on the last repetitions is what puts size and shape on your thighs.

Squats: Free Weights or Cybex Machine: Warm-up with light weights, then do 4 sets of 6 to 3 reps. Squats both back and front also develop the gluts which is covered in the next body part. Use the "two pair of pants method" or tight fitting jeans so the squats won't hurt your knees and low back.

Front Squats: Place the bar in front of your neck and cross your arms to support it. This works the front portion of the thighs. Do two Squat /Quad Extension Super-sets if you have access to a quad machine.

The following exercises are if you work-out at a gym and want more ways to develop the legs.

Quad Extension, Machine or Leg weights: If you don't have access to a leg extension machine then use strap-on Velcro leg weights. Start light then add weight. Hold the extended position and contract the leg firmly. Do sets of 12-20 reps or whatever it takes to reach muscle failure. Start very light and keep adding weight and then come down again until the quads really burn. This will bring out the definition in the two muscles above the knee.

Super-set Quad Extensions with front squats. A Super-set is when you do one exercise to the maximum or to muscle failure and then without any rest do a another different, related exercise to force even more blood in the muscles which stimulates them to grow.

Leg Press Machine: On this machine you sit down with your bent legs up to your chest and then you extend them. Start light and then add weight. 2-3 sets of 6-8 reps.

Glut Machine: Glut machines isolate the gluteus maximus and minimus. Start light and raise the weight until you can only do 3 reps.

Inner Thigh Machine: Use a weight heavy enough to feel a burn after doing 4 to 6 reps. These can be done with leg weights also.

Outer Thigh Machine: Works the outer gluts also. Use a weight heavy enough to do 6 to 8 reps. Can be done with leg weights.

Calf Exercises

AT HOME: Do one legged toe raises on a board or step while holding a dumbbell. Running also develops the calves.

GYM: Leg Press Machine: Using a heavy weight hold the contracted position to really work the calves. Super-set this with the following two exercises. **Seated Calf Machine:** Again hold the contracted position to really isolate the calves. **Standing Calf Machine:** Use a heavy weight in order to gain size and hold and contract at the top. Do 6 to 8 reps in order to really make the calves burn and fail to contract. You can work calves at every workout just like abdominals.

GLUTS

To develop the gluts, short for the gluteal muscles also known as the buttocks, squats including back, front and hack is the best exercise. In addition the following are also useful:

1. Running or walking fast up hills or stairs will develop the gluts.

2. Leg weights strapped to the legs are also excellent. Kneel on your knees on a pad, sofa or bed and shoot back the bended leg as far as possible and hold it for a second or two. Follow this keeping the knee straight and extend the leg and hold. Then stand up and supported against a wall extend the leg back with the knee kept straight.

3. The "lunge" is done by walking in a straight line. A long stride is taken and the other knee touches the ground lightly and then comes up. Keep lunging up and down the room until your legs and butt can't do anymore. Use light weight dumbbells in each hand if you need extra weight.

4. Straight-leg dead lift using a light weight. Works hamstrings and gluts.

Glut Machines: There are machines at the gym that isolate the gluts.

1. One of them has you leaning over on a pad with your leg cocked to shoot back a weighted foot holder. Hold the extended position if possible to feel the gluts work.

2. Another machine has a padded rod that you put your leg over catching it behind the knee and then you force it back using your buttock muscles. Most gyms have a weighted cable pulley system and a leg strap that you can put on your ankle. With a straight leg extend back to work the gluts.

SHOULDERS

Military Press: Military barbell presses are excellent for developing mass. Press the barbell overhead. Upright rowers to develop the trapezius muscles above the shoulders are done by holding a barbell with your hands close together and pulling it up to the chin then lowering it slowly. During the lighter weights one can do the front shoulder lift holding the bar at shoulder width and lifting it over the head with locked elbows.

Dumbbell Press: With the dumbbell weights or the weights designed to be grasped in the hand do the seated dumbbell shoulder press sitting down on a comfortable bench/chair or standing and pushing the dumbbells over head doing 2 to 3 sets of 3 to 6 reps. This develops the front and side shoulder.

Dumbbell Superset:
Follow the above heavy presses with the following dumbbell superset.

1. First do bent over dumbbells for the rear delts. This is done by taking light weight dumbbells and bending over, then keep the elbows locked and lift and hold, feeling the rear deltoids. Next take a lightweight dumbbell and lift it sideways, keeping the elbow locked until it is above the head slightly and hold it then lower and do 6 reps on each side.

2. Next do lateral raises using both dumbbells and moving them out to the side and holding momentarily, the elbows are bent.

3. Then without rest do front lifts holding the elbows stiff and lift the weights to eye level one dumbbell at a time. Start with a light weight doing 6-8 repetitions and then move up until you can do just 1 to 3 repetitions or "reps". This is the pyramid method of starting light and going as heavy as you can, doing just one rep. At the higher weights rest between sets until refreshed and ready to do another set.

Trapezius Exercises:

1. **Barbell shrugs:** to develop the trapezius are done by grabbing the bar at shoulder length and shrugging the shoulders and holding for 3 seconds. It can also be done holding the bar behind you and with dumbbells. On the last rep of your hack squats use the heavy weight and shrug and hold as many times as you can. Heavy behind the back shrugs really develop the traps.

2. **Upright rowers:** Grab a barbell with two hands and a close grip. Bring the barbell up to chin level and then lower slowly. Again use the pyramid system, starting light and adding weight.

BICEPS

1. **Standing barbell curls:** Warm up with light weight and quickly move up to the most weight you can do for 3 to 1 repetitions.

2. **Dumbbell curls,** superset with dumbbell reverse curls and wrist curls which develops the forearm. Do 2 sets.

3. **Concentration curls:** Done bent over at the waist with arm hanging down and then moving dumbbell to the chin position and holding. Do 2 sets on each arm.

4. **Pull-ups:** using a palms toward you grip which isolates the biceps. Do as many as possible. On the last few reps come down as slowly as you can.

Remember: to keep the body and mind youthful you must exercise to prevent the loss of your shape. Weightlifting is the best exercise to gain muscle mass.

TRICEPS

1. **Close grip barbell bench press:** Grip the bar a little closer than your shoulders. Use as heavy a weight as needed to do just 6 repetitions. One to two sets.

2. **Barbell triceps pull-overs using a bar:** Lie on your back on a bench, bed or stool and hang over the edge and grab the bar over your head with bent elbows. Then bring the bar overhead feeling the triceps as you do the movement. Use enough weight to just barely do 6 reps.

3. **Triceps push downs on the machine:** Grab the rope attachment and push down using the triceps with a straight back. 1 to 2 good sets of 6-8 reps.

4. **Dumbbell triceps isolation:** Take one lightweight dumbbell and bend your elbow so the weight starts at the back of the head, then straighten the elbow overhead. 1 or 2 sets using enough weight to do 4-6 reps.

WEIGHT LIFTING IS THE BEST EXERCISE TO KEEP THE MUSCLES IN SHAPE

Intensive lifting done 2-3 times per week is all that is needed. Working in the garden; planting, digging, pruning, watering, fertilizing is a good form of exercise but it does not isolate certain muscle groups like weight lifting does. Weight lifting will make your body look in shape and it has also been proven to help your energy power centers, the mitochondria stay young and fit.

CHEST

1. **Bench press with a barbell:** wide grip, medium grip and close grip. The wide grip widens the chest, the middle grip works the middle muscles and the close grip defines the inner chest and triceps. Lie on a bench press on your back and lift off the weight from the rack, then lower the barbell to your chest and press it until your elbows are straight.

Use heavier weight and 3 to 6 repetitions to add size to the chest and lighter weight and 8 to 20 reps to define the chest.

2. **Bench press with dumbbells:** First do a fly type press (with locked elbows move dumbbells out to sides and back), followed by the regular bench press right after. 2 sets of 6 to 8 reps.

3. **Incline bench press:** Works the upper part of the chest, the front shoulder and the whole shoulder. A decline bench press works to define the bottom of the chest.

If your chest is naturally well developed and large in size, just do incline presses to work the shoulders more and wide, medium and close hand position push-ups to keep it well defined.

4. **Pull-overs with straight arms:** Develops the upper and lower part of the chest. Also gives thickness and striations. It also widens the back to give a V-shape.

BACK

1. **Rowers with dumbbells:** Take one dumbbell and bend over at the waist with one knee on a bench, chair or bed then pull the weight up to the chest. Then repeat with the other arm. This avoids injury to the low back.

2. **Rowers with barbell:** Using a very lightweight barbell and a wide grip, bend over at the waist, extend the arms then pull up the barbell to the chest and lower slowly.

3. **Pull ups:** Are great for the upper back if you have a bar or a tree branch nearby. You can pull up so the bar goes behind your neck in addition to pulling up to the chin. A wider grip widens the back.

STOMACH, WAIST AND LOWER BACK

The most important part in creating a trim waist is the diet. If you eat too much without burning it off with exercise, then fat will form around the waist and stomach. The waist and stomach are the body's storage depot. Again, if we eat more than we can burn off during the day (especially fat-rich foods like cheese, cream), fat will form.

Eating heavy later at night will just pad your waistline. Fats, cooked starches and bread tend to form fat the quickest, but even excess banana and papaya will form fat and it all goes right to the stomach and waist. If you get constipated, this will make the waistline expand, making you look fat. Eating plenty of sweet fruit, blended aloe vera and juiced raw, green leafy, starchless vegetables will keep you regular and unconstipated.

The midsection or your core, with a flat hard stomach, lean waist and strong back is very important for a fit physique. A superset doing one exercise after the other without rest really works the midsection.

First do:
1. Sit-ups with a light weight plate (with your feet held under the barbell or under a bed or sofa), then do them without weight, then do

2. Bicycle crunches done by slowly bringing one knee to the opposite elbow alternating legs, then do

3. Crunches or lifting the head and shoulders off the ground looking up with bent knee holding as long as you can in the contracted position, then do

4. Leg-ups lifting the legs up in the air while slightly bending the knees, then right after do

5. Leg-ups holding the contracted position of the legs about 6 inches above the floor, with your hands under your waist to give you support, hold until failure occurs.

The oblique muscles are on the side of the waist. The best way to exercise these muscles is to place a broomstick behind your neck and rotate it so it's pointed straight ahead, then rotate it to the other side picking up speed as you go until you feel a burn in the muscles which is usually about 100-200 reps. It can even be done watching television.

Really feel the rotation and flex the side muscles as you do them. This twisting exercise can also be done with weight. Take a ten or five pound weight and hold it in both hands, then rotate until your shoulders are facing front to back then rotate to the other side. Do 15-25 repetitions.

Another good exercise for the side waist is holding a light weight dumbbell or plate (5-20 pounds) in one hand and leaning to the side stretching, then return to the upright. These exercises really firm up the "love handle area".

The low back is worked by doing back contractions lying on a bench or bed and contracting the back up and holding. Or light weights can be held behind the neck while standing and then lowering your head to the waist level and then returning.

Working out will get the endorphin hormones to kick in and that will get you feeling blissful. Endorphin means literally "morphine within", derived from the words endogenous morphine, the true and natural opiate of the people. Depression can occur from the lack of it. Cultivate endorphins through exercise, diet, laughing and massage.

EXAMPLE ROUTINES 30-40 MINUTES
3 TIMES PER WEEK OR EVERY OTHER DAY

The four major body parts are:
1. Legs, Calves
2. Shoulders: trapezius, side, front and rear deltoids
3. Chest and Back
4. Arms: triceps, biceps, forearms
You can combine all of them and do a full body workout doing only one or two exercises for each body part, or you can do a whole body workout once a week using heavy weights and then do lighter lifting on your weak areas for the other days. **Abdominals and obliques (side waist muscles) are done after or before each workout**. Run sprints uphill or walk fast uphill before working out enough to feel your legs get pumped and your heart rate racing.

1. Legs:
Run or walk uphill fast to warm-up
Back squats, Front squats, Leg extension machine, Leg curl machine

Hack squats
Calves: One foot calve raises with/without dumbbell, Calf machines; standing, seated, leg press

2. Shoulders:
Military press with barbell, Barbell behind the neck presses
Dumbbell presses
Dumbbell and cable rear deltoid, front deltoid, side deltoid, see shoulder section for how to do these exercises

3. Chest and Back:
Incline press or bench press with barbell or dumbbells, Push-ups, Pull-ups, One arm bent over rowers with dumbbell

4. Arms:
Close grip bench press/ superset with triceps press and pullovers using barbell
One arm triceps press using dumbbell
Forearm reverse curls with barbell/ superset with barbell curls
Wrist curls with barbell
Dumbbell curls/ superset with dumbbell reverse curls
Concentration dumbbell curls
Pull-ups reversed to isolate the biceps

Working out every other day gives your muscles a chance to recuperate. Overtraining and training everyday stresses your body making it release the stress hormones cortisol and human growth hormone. Working out every other day makes you want to workout when the time comes because your body is rested. Try a whole body workout doing less exercises for each body part and see how it feels. Use different exercises for the same body part on the following workout.

MAKE THE WEEKLY COMMITMENT

Knowing it's a short (30-40 minutes), hard workout every other day will keep you consistent. If you are really busy make sure you get at least one good workout in per week doing weights and cardio. Going two weeks without weights can make your muscles go flaccid and lose size and strength. Get started today on a new life of exercise which will give you a new body and a new mind, full of strength and beauty like the classic Greek ideal; a sound mind in a sound body.

THE HEALING
POWER OF FRUIT

HOW FRUIT ORCHARDING
CAN HELP SAVE OUR PLANET

Fruit is the food that can best feed the world; with the highest acreage yield (400,000 lbs. per acre) according to the Fruitarian Network (2003). Dr. Miklos Faust, former chief of the USDA fruit labs points out that centenarian apple trees can drop 2 tons (each) of food. Linear, two dimensional crop rows of vegetables, beans or grains cannot compete with a tree that grows upward and spherically in three dimensions.

By creating fruit forests or orchard gardens to supply our food we can help stabilize the climate since trees convert the greenhouse gas CO_2 to oxygen and plant fiber. Forests bring rain to deserts and drought areas through the evaporation of large amounts of water. They also absorb noise, filter the air, produce healthful negative ions and create a peaceful environment.

A fruit grove or orchard also provides a habitat for wild animals. The most healthy and ecological fast food is fruit. Fruit even comes with its own packaging, eliminating waste.

AN APPLE A DAY, OR BETTER YET 2 OR
MORE APPLES A DAY KEEPS THE DOCTOR AWAY

Benjamin Franklin, a vegetarian, coined the phrase, "An apple a day keeps the doctor away." Apple, known as the Fruit of the Gods, is a very powerful source of spiritual energy that encourages balance and harmony according to D. W. Hauck (1998) at the alchemylab.com website.

In ancient Greece and Rome, apples were eaten at Diana's Festival (August 13). The Egyptians offered apples to their highest and most powerful priests, whom they considered guardians of hidden knowledge.

In the Middle Ages sliced apples were used to foretell the future and eating them regularly was said to enable a person to live over 200 years. Modern clinical studies have proven that eating apples reduces cancer risk. Apples are quite a versatile food what with apple sauce, apple juice, apple cider and apple pie.

THE HEALTH BENEFITS OF APPLES

They have been called the "King of Fruits" and they also may be the king of disease prevention or keeping the doctor away.

The fiber in apples is mostly soluble fiber, called pectin, which has a successful record as a cholesterol reducer going back to research in the early 1960s. Apples rank near the top among fruits and vegetables as a source of pectin, providing .78 grams per 100 grams of the edible portion of fruit. Apples are also a delicious source of dietary fiber; a medium apple contains about five grams of fiber, more than most cereals.

Apples also contain important flavonoids. Flavonoids are naturally-occurring plant compounds that have antioxidant properties. Apples have the highest concentration of flavonoids of any fruit. 100 grams of unpeeled fresh apple, about two-thirds of a medium-sized apple, provides the total antioxidant activity of 1,500 milligrams of vitamin C. A Finnish study (Knekt, Jarvinen, Reunanen, & Maatela, 1996) published in the prestigious British Medical Journal showed that people who eat a diet rich in flavonoids have a lower incidence of heart disease. Other studies indicate that flavonoids may help prevent strokes. Naturally grown apples are best which means without artificial pesticides or fertilizers which can cause headache, nerve problems and nutritional imbalances.

THE HEALING PROPERTIES
OF CHERRIES

Cherries have long been praised for their health benefits, but now this has new scientific evidence to prove it. A researcher in the study of melatonin discovered the disease fighting antioxidant in red tart cherries. This is the first time melatonin has been found as a naturally occurring substance in food.

Russell J. Reiter, professor of neuroendocrinology at The University of Texas Health Science Center in San Antonio, said results of the five-month study show that melatonin is present in substantial quantities in tart cherries and that "Studies have shown that melatonin is beneficial for slowing the aging process, promoting sleep and helping with the effects of jet lag."

The same chemicals that give tart cherries their color may relieve pain better than aspirin and ibuprofen. Melatonin, it turns out is one of the most potent antioxidants known to man. Cherries in fresh and dried form would be the most natural way to augment the anti-oxidant level of the body. Cherries may provide antioxidant protection comparable to commercially available supplements such as vitamin E and vitamin C. The capuli or Andean mountain cherry, if properly cultivated, can be sweet, yet not overly sweet and not acidic like some temperate cherries. It's in season for 5-6 months. At one time the inter-Andean plateau was forested with capuli trees. The Spanish colonists used the hardwood of the capuli to build their churches and residences and thus the wild, virgin, native forests were cut down.

THE HEALING PROPERTIES OF GRAPES

Grapes are chock full of phytonutrients such as resveratrol, quercetin, anthocyanin and catechin. Resveratrol, found primarily in the skin of grapes, has been found in preliminary studies to fight breast, liver and colon cancers. Resveratrol is also believed to play a role in the reduction of heart disease and has been shown to exhibit anti-inflammatory properties. Dr. John Harvey Kellogg, (his brother created Kellogg's corn flakes), back in 1870 at his famous clinic in Battlecreek, Michigan would prescribe 10 to 14 pounds of grapes per day to cure patients of high blood pressure. For those with heart problems it was grapes and more grapes and for skinny patients he advised 26 feedings a day to gain weight. In 1928 Dr. Johanna Brandt, a South African naturopath, published a book called "The Grape Cure" after having an illumination and taught that grapes could cure most every disease including cancer.

HEALING BLUEBERRIES
THE NUMBER #1 ANTIOXIDANT

Blueberries are number one in anti-oxidant activity according to the findings of USDA scientists Dr. Ronald Prior and Dr. Guohuacao from the Jean Mayer Human Nutrition Research Centre on Aging at Tufts University. Flavonoids, including anthocyanins, are responsible for the intense blue color of wild blueberries which contain the highest food source of antioxidants known. Antioxidants prevent cell damage due to oxidation by free radicals and thus prevent cancer and many age related diseases such as the loss of memory and motor skills.

Of all the fruits tested, wild blueberries showed the greatest anti-cancer activity according to Dr. Mary Ann Smith of the University of Illinois and is due to the flavonoids they contain. Dr. Richard Passwater, Ph.D., research director at Maryland's Solgar Nutritional Research Center says proanthocyanoidins (PACs) produce the intense color of blueberries, huckleberries, plums and purple or red grapes. PACs strengthen the blood capillaries which result in less constriction of veins which could lead to swollen feet or ankles. They also aid rapid healing of bruises and well developed collagen creating fewer wrinkles and less swollen or varicose veins. Blueberries, huckleberries, black and red raspberries, boysenberries, blackberries and strawberries are the fruits highest in fiber and phyto-nutrients and the lowest in sugar.

In a study published in the Nutritional Neuroscience journal (2004) by Casadesus G. et al., a blueberry-supplemented diet was found to greatly enhance the memory of laboratory animals.

When later studied in vitro, the animals' brains demonstrated structural changes associated with an improved capacity for learning. Researchers believe the two findings are directly related.

Research published in the journal Neurobiology of Aging (2005) by Lau F. C. et al. showed that nutritional antioxidants found in blueberries can reverse age-related declines in neuronal signal transfer as well as cognitive and motor deficits.

The investigators speculated that blueberry supplementation may also help slow declines in brain function that accompany diseases such as Alzheimer's disease and Parkinson's disease.

This is wonderful news for those of us over 50 who start to forget things more and more as the years pass. This can be very disturbing with a sense of loss of control of your life. By adding blueberries to our diet we can help the loss of memory and brain power.

In an study published in Biochemistry and Cell Biology (2005) Matchett M. D. et al found that 24 hours of exposure to extracts of blueberry antioxidants sharply reduced the production of matrix metalloproteinases—enzymes believed to play key roles in malignant tissue metastasis—in human prostate cancer cells.

This led the researchers to postulate that blueberry supplementation may help prevent tumor metastasis.

In other words blueberries can help prevent cancer cells and in particular those that want to spread and crowd out other beneficial cells. It's nice to know that there are foods like blueberries that are known to make cancer cells benign.

CAROB

The pod of the carob tree is technically a legume and not a fruit. Most fruits have high water content of usually 80% but the carob pod is only 3.58% water. Mixed with fresh mashed banana, dried carob powder becomes moist and water rich like most other fruits.

The value in this "legume-fruit" is that it is very high in calcium and other important minerals. Carob powder contains 348 milligrams calcium and 79 milligrams phosphorus per 100 grams or about one cup (103 grams). This ratio is important because if phosphorus is in a higher proportion than calcium then the calcium will not be absorbed. Carob is also high in copper (.59 milligrams per cup) which has been linked to helping restore the natural color of the hair.

One way to eat raw carob powder is to mix it with ripe bananas, mashing it with a fork. You can add it to blended papaya and banana for a more moist end product. A moister consistency is desired because the powder is water poor and thus is more digestible when moist.

During World War II food shortages forced the Greek people to eat carob bread because there was no wheat flour available. Carob is also known as St. John's Bread. Locusts was mistranslated in the Bible because the locust bean tree is the carob tree. John the Baptist ate the wild carob pods whole in the desert. Carob is high in the minerals calcium and magnesium which are crucial in maintaining strong teeth and bones.

THE GLYCEMIC INDEX

The Glycemic Index or GI will guide you in choosing foods that don't raise the blood sugar excessively thus avoiding insulin over-secretion and its negative effects. The Glycemic Index is a numerical system of measuring how fast a carbohydrate triggers a rise in circulating blood sugar. The higher the number, the greater the blood sugar response. Insulin raises homocysteine levels which is implicated in causing heart disease.

Insulin resistance means your cells become unable to use insulin to lower blood sugar or glucose due to a past history of constant overdose of excess secretion of insulin which makes them less responsive. One symptom of this condition is fatigue after eating or a short time after eating. Certain fruits are high on the list like dates, over-ripe bananas and watermelon and need to be eaten in moderation.

Glucose is approximately the index of 100

FRUIT AND FRUIT PRODUCTS
Cherries 22
Strawberry 25
Raspberry 25
Blackberry, mulberry 25
Grapefruit 25
Apricots, dried 31
Pear, fresh 37
Apple 38
Plum 39
Apple juice 41
Peach, fresh 42
Orange 44
Pear, canned 44
Grapes 46
Pineapple juice 46
Peach, canned 47
Grapefruit juice 48
Orange juice 52
Kiwifruit 53
Banana 54
Note: A 1992 study by Hermansen et al. reported that the GI for underripe bananas was 43 and that for overripe bananas was 74. In underripe bananas the starch constitutes 80-90 percent of the carbohydrate content, which as the banana ripens, changes to free sugars. Overripe bananas are too sweet and if underripe are too starchy. When the brown spots first appear is the precise time to eat the banana.

Fruit cocktail 55
Mango 56
Sultanas 56
Apricots, fresh 57
Pawpaw or papaya 58
Apricots, canned, syrup 64
Raisins 64 (raisins have the same GI as white sugar)
Rock melon (muskmelon, cantaloupe) 65
Pineapple 66 (notice the juice is only 46)
Watermelon 72
Dates 103

SUGARS
Sucrose White sugar 64
Fructose 22 (low GI but really a toxic refined chemical)
Lactose 46
Honey 58
High fructose corn syrup 62

FOODS FOR COMPARISON:
Potato, baked 85
Wheat bread, white 71
Rice, brown 55
Rice, wild, Saskatchewan 57
Rice, white 58
High Fiber Rye Crisp bread 65
Yogurt, unspecified 36

Carrot juice quality depends on the carrot variety, soil and cultivation practices. California carrots are known to be much sweeter than others. Straight carrot juice not mixed with other green vegetables has a high GI.

Some fruits are not too be eaten alone because they are too sweet and sugary. You can tell by the feeling you get after eating them, getting a strong sugar rush then a big crash. Cherimoyas are a case in point. You could eat cherimoyas, then eat some apples and cherries to balance the high sugar content. Low GI fruits will dilute the effect of the high sugar content of the cherimoyas.

Dates have a very high GI (above 100) and need to be eaten in moderation. The more tart or acid the fruit, like cherries, berries, crisp apples and citrus, the lower the GI.

APPENDIX

HOME REMEDIES FOR CANCER

UCLA researchers (Mori et al., 2006) shrank tumors by 80% with the heat from habanero peppers. That is quite extraordinary in terms of what is usually accomplished with toxic drugs. The study conducted at Cedars Sinai Medical Center in Los Angeles, California, USA in collaboration with UCLA Doctors and researchers, concluded that an ingredient known as capsaicin, found in habanero peppers, had the ability to make prostate cancer cells commit suicide. Capsaicin is also found in the jalapeno pepper, but the habanero has the highest content of capsaicin. The study, conducted with mice, manifested approximately an 80% decrease in prostate tumor size versus untreated mice.

The State of New Mexico has the lowest cancer mortality rate of all 50 states. They probably eat more peppers in New Mexico per capita than all the other states. Mexico has the 167th lowest cancer (all cancers) death rate out of 192 countries; 81.5 per 100,000.

Kelley Eidem's stage four cancer success in curing himself with habaneras peppers preceded the UCLA researchers by seven years, and he didn't shrink his tumors by 80%, he shrank them 100%.

He smothered one grated habanero pepper with seeds and two cloves of grated garlic with butter putting them on bread each day. He also used cod liver oil, but that is not recommended because it can cause heart attacks (Veierød, Thelle, & Laake, 1997).

The UCLA researchers just used habanero peppers without the cod liver oil and accomplished an 80% reduction in cancer tumors. UCLA's research results confirmed this method was an extremely powerful weapon against cancer.

In another more recent corroborating study, conducted at the University of Pittsburgh Medical School (Zhang, Humphreys, Sahu, Shi, & Srivastava, 2008) capsaicin was shown to have induced apoptosis (cellular suicide) of pancreatic cancer cells. Researchers said, " ... results of the study show that capsaicin is an effective inhibitor of in vitro (test tube) and in vivo (in living organisms) growth of pancreatic cancer cells."

Don Imus is now trying to keep trouble away by putting "hot stuff into his mouth" in the form of habanero peppers, in his ongoing effort to manage and fight prostate cancer.

Dr. Lee used progesterone cream to cure prostate cancer in his patients. Aspirin has been proven clinically to reduce cancer risk.

Dr. Raymond Peat, who first told Dr. Lee about progesterone, says about progesterone, "It has been used quite a bit for kidney, lung, and prostate cancers. The brain has a high concentration of it naturally, so it's probably helpful there, too. With the right preparation, it could probably be used effectively in the stomach, colon, and bladder. I know of a couple of instances where it helped pancreas cancer. High doses of aspirin, with vitamin K, are helpful for any kind of cancer. The diet should emphasize fruit, milk, and cheese."

FRUIT CLASSIFICATION CHART ACCORDING TO TRADITIONAL CHINESE MEDICINE

Fruit, according to Chinese Traditional Medicine, should be eaten primarily during the warm and hot seasons.

During the cold season, highly cooling fruit such as bananas, oranges and lemons should be avoided to prevent developing cold in the body.

To treat a person who is overly yin; often tired and exhausted, introverted in personality, has a weak pulse and cold hands, give red/purple grapes, peaches, plums and cherries.

An overly yang person would benefit from apple, citrus, pineapple and tangerine.

Apple
Thermal nature: Cool to Cold
Flavor: Sweet and sour
Organ: Stomach, spleen, lung
Element: Earth, wood
Effect: Clears heat, relieves agitation, alleviates summer heat, creates body fluids, moistens the lung, relieves diarrhea, stimulates appetite. Creates body fluids, moistens lung, quenches thirst and

relieves cough.

Nutrients: Highest fruit in flavonoids, malic acid, pectin Very high in minerals and trace elements, iron especially.

Indications: Raw apple is good following excess alcohol consumption. In a overly yin condition take grated apple slightly heated or as a cooked fruit compote or apple sauce.

Apricot
Thermal nature: Neutral to warm
Flavor: Sweet and sour
Organ: Stomach, lung
Indications: Due to their high iron content and warming effect, apricots are recommended during pregnancy. Eaten to excess, can damage teeth.

Banana
Thermal nature: Cold
Flavor: Sweet
Organ: Stomach, large intestine
Element: Earth
Effect: Clears heat, enriches yin, moistens and detoxifies intestines, creates body fluids, moistens stomach.
Nutrients: Contains serotonin the good mood hormone. High in pantothenic acid and folic acid. High in potassium which is good for the heart.
Indications: Raw bananas recommended for constipation and bleeding hemorrhoids. Not recommended for cold and overly yin conditions or with excess mucus.

Cherry
Thermal nature: Warm
Flavor: Sweet
Organ: Stomach, spleen (liver and kidney)
Element: Earth
Effect: Supplements the center burner, qi, and blood; supplements and moistens liver and spleen, disperses blood stasis.
Nutrients: Iron, B1, B2, B3
Indications: Coldness, exhaustion, fatigue, insomnia, weakness and pain in the knees and hips.

Grape
Thermal nature: Neutral
Flavor: Sweet and sour

Organ: Spleen, lung, kidneys (liver)
Element: Wood and earth
Effect: Supplements kidneys and liver, supplements qi, promotes blood formation, creates body fluids, strengthens muscles, sinews and bones; diuretic.
Nutrients: Rich in glucose, highest potassium content in fruit, iron, copper, calcium, bioflavonoids, resveratrol. Raisins are higher in carbohydrate, iron and calcium than fresh grapes.
Indications: Weakness and pain in spine, knees and hips, frailty.

Grapefruit
Thermal nature: Cool to cold, peel warm.
Flavor: Sweet and sour, peel sweet and bitter.
Organ: Stomach, lung, peel; stomach-kidney-gallbladder
Element: Earth
Effect: Flesh: creates body fluids, relieves thirst. Peel: stomach-kidney-gallbladder.
Nutrients: Vitamin C.
Indications: Bronchitis with yellow-green mucus, excessive alcohol consumption

Mango
Thermal nature: Neutral
Flavor: Sweet, sour
Organ: Stomach, lung
Element: Earth
Effect: Regenerates body fluids, stops cough, stops thirst, strengthens stomach
Nutrients: Vitamin A, magnesium, chlorine, niacin
Indications: Cough, thirst, poor digestion, enlarged prostate.

Orange
Thermal nature: Cooling
Flavor: Sweet, sour
Organ: Lungs, Spleen, Stomach
Element: Earth
Effect: Lubricates lungs, resolves mucus, strengthens spleen increases appetite, quenches thirst, promotes body fluids.
Nutrients: Vitamin C, bioflavonoids, citric acid.
Indications: Thirst, dehydration, stagnant chi, hernia.

Papaya
Thermal nature: Neutral

Flavor: Sweet
Organ: Heart, lungs, bladder
Element: Earth
Effect: Strengthens stomach and spleen, digestion, clears summer heat, lubricates lungs, stops cough, aids irritability, kills worms, increases milk production.
Nutrients: Vitamin A, vitamin C, potassium.
Indications: Cough, indigestion, stomach ache, eczema, skin lesions, intestinal worms.

Peach
Thermal nature: Warm to hot
Flavor: Sweet-sour
Organ: Stomach, large intestine, (liver).
Element: Earth, metal, wood
Effect: Creates body fluids, moistens intestines, moves blood, dissolves blood stasis, can soften hardness.
Nutrients: Very good potassium-sodium ratio, zinc.
Indications: Constipation especially in elderly people.

Pear
Thermal nature: Cool
Flavor: Sweet
Organ: Lung, stomach
Element: Wood, earth
Effect: Clears heat, moistens dryness, creates body fluids, transforms phlegm
Nutrients: Especially rich in potassium, hormone-like substances.
Indications: Irritated, hoarse vocal chords, loss of voice, dry cough, constipation.

Plum
Thermal nature: Neutral to warm
Flavor: Sweet and sour
Organ: Liver, kidney, stomach
Element: Earth, wood, water
Effect: Clears liver heat, disperses qi stagnation and blood stasis, creates body fluids, diuretic.
Nutrients: Rich in iron, Excellent K-Na and Ca-P ratio
Indications: Liver stagnation and heat, tendency to outbursts of rage, restlessness, irritability, night sweat.

Pineapple
Thermal nature: Neutral to cool
Flavor: Sweet and sour
Organ: Stomach, gallbladder
Element: Earth
Effect: Disperses summer heat, creates body fluids, thirst-quenching, diuretic, promotes digestion.
Nutrients: Bromelain enzyme promotes digestion of protein, iron, copper, zinc.
Indications: Thirst, dry mouth, nausea, lack of appetite, restlessness.

Strawberry
Thermal nature: Cooling
Flavor: Sweet, sour
Organ: Lungs, spleen, stomach
Element: Metal, Earth
Effect: Lubricates lungs, promotes body fluids, strengthens spleen, detoxifies alcohol intoxication.
Nutrients: Silicon, iron, vitamin C.
Indications: Dry cough, sore throat, difficult urination, food retention, lack of appetite.

Watermelon
Thermal nature: Cold
Flavor: Sweet
Organ: Kidney, bladder
Element: Water, Earth
Effect: Quenches thirst, relieves irritability, dispels summer heat problems, promotes diuresis, detoxifies.
Nutrients: Vitamin A, bromine, potassium.
Indications: Sores, dry mouth, summer heat irritability, jaundice, edema, difficult urination, bloody dysentery.

For someone who eats a diet with a large percentage of fruit, it's wise to eat fruits that are warming and neutral to balance the majority of fruits which are cool or cold.

Peach is the only hot fruit, cherries are warm, plums and apricot are neutral to warming. Grapes are listed as neutral but red and purple grapes are indicated as warming foods. Papaya and mango are neutral fruits. Pineapple is neutral to cool. Watermelon and bananas are the only cold fruits listed, while the rest of them are cool to cooling.

To eat a lot of cool to cold apples during the cold winter months would make your body too yin and cold.

Carob powder, though not listed, has a warming effect. Papaya, a neutral fruit, is available during the winter.

Steamed kabocha squash is a good choice during the cold winter months in temperate regions.

THE YIN AND YANG OF FOODS

Eating mostly Yin foods causes the body to produce only Yin energy, which is darker, slower-moving and has a pacifying effect. It gives a feeling of lightness, making the body less full and cooler.

Eating predominantly Yang foods causes the body to produce only Yang energy, which is faster, hotter and much more energetic. Yang foods boost mental strength and encourage assertive and aggressive behaviors.

The best way to good health is to choose foods that are balanced, containing both Yin and Yang energies. Foods that are mostly Yin or Yang should be treated with caution.

Those who are excessively passive or wishy-washy, disorganized, lazy or apathetic, need to eat more Yang energy foods. For those with rigid thinking patterns and driven personalities, the Yin energy foods will help to restore balance.

Yin Alkaline Forming Foods: Cocoa, fruit juices, coffee, tea, mineral water, soda water and well water, honey, mustard, ginger, pepper, curry, cinnamon, tropical fruits, dates, figs, lemons, grapes, bananas, peaches, currants, pears, plums, oranges, watermelon, apples, cherries, strawberries, potatoes, eggplant, tomatoes, shiitake, taro, potatoes, cucumber, sweet potatoes, mushrooms, spinach, asparagus, broccoli, celery, cabbage, pumpkin, onions, turnips, daikon, nori, hijiki, carrots.

Yin Acid Forming Foods: Most chemicals, vinegar, saccharin, vodka, some wine, whiskey, sake, beer, soybeans, green peas, tofu, white beans, pinto beans, black beans, chickpeas, red beans (azuki), macaroni, spaghetti, cashews, peanuts, almonds, chestnuts, corn oil, olive oil, peanut butter, sesame butter.

Yang Alkaline Forming Foods: Dandelion tea, mu tea, ginseng, millet, soy sauce, miso, umeboshi, salt, wakame, kombu, lotus root, burdock, dandelion root.

Yang Acid Forming Foods: Cornmeal, oats, barley, rye, wheat, rice, buckwheat, shellfish, eel, carp, white meat fish, cheese, fowl, meat, tuna, salmon, eggs and cow's milk.

According to the Tao of food, balanced Yin and Yang energy foods are: grains, seeds, rice, root vegetables, cheese and apples.

The acid forming and alkaline forming foods can be classified Yin or Yang according to their sodium, potassium, calcium, magnesium phosphorus and sulfur content. Yin acid forming foods are high in phosphorus and sulfur, and at the same time are low in sodium. Yang acid forming foods are high in phosphorus, sulfur and sodium. Yin alkaline forming foods are high in potassium, calcium and low in phosphorus and sulfur. Yang alkaline forming foods are high in sodium, magnesium and low in phosphorus and sulfur.

Eating what is locally grown helps keep your body balanced with the local climate. For example, if you lived in the tropics you would eat the Yin energy fruits such as pineapple, figs, papaya, banana and mango. These Yin energy foods combat the heat of the Yang tropical climate. The heat in tropical climates (Yang) being balanced by the watery fruits (Yin) that grow there. Tropical fruits support the expansion of pores to keep the body cool. If tropical fruits (Yin) are eaten in a Winter climate (Yin), the person often feels too cold (Yin). Likewise, in colder climates it is beneficial to eat very warming Yang energy foods, such as cooked vegetables.

Disorders can be classified by their Yin / Yang balance.
Excess Yin Foods; Leukemia, Meningitis, Colitis, Epilepsy, Emphysema, Diabetes, Asthma, Skin cancer, Hypersensitivity, Nervousness. Excess Yang Foods; Jaundice, Gout, Ulcers, Tongue cancer, Lung cancer, Pancreatic cancer, Kidney cancer, Colon cancer, Muscular dystrophy, Anger, Paranoia. Excess Yin & Yang; Arteriosclerosis, Hepatitis, Uremia, Gallstones, Breast cancer, Uterine cancer, Bladder cancer, Schizophrenia.

When we digest "dead" food, which lacks frequency, life force, or what is commonly known as ch'i energy, we feel sluggish and lethargic. Examples of dead foods are: old, wilted, overly refrigerated vegetables and green, unripe or old fruit.

Processed and refined foods lack life energy or chi and fill our bodies with chemicals and toxins that block energy flow. In Ayurvedic medicine, the traditional medical system of India, these dead, putrid foods are called Tamasic and leave you tired and sluggish as opposed to the Sattvic foods like fresh fruits and yogurt that leave you calm and alert. Rajasic foods, like meat, leave one agitated and restless.

THE pH OF FRUITS AND VEGETABLES

The pH value of a food tells us how acidic it is. 7 is neutral in the pH scale. Anything lower than this will be more and more acidic as the numbers get lower. Above pH 7 means the food is alkaline.

Foods like pineapple and citrus fruits like oranges and tangerines are lower on the pH scale; around 3 to 4. Most vegetables are around 5 to 7. Pineapple juice is acidic, pH 3.30 - 3.60 and therefore it can erode the enamel of the teeth causing damage. The same applies to orange juice because it has a pH value between 3.30 and 4.19. Green pineapples or oranges will give even more acidic juices which can erode tooth enamel and inside the body can drain the calcium reserve stored in the teeth and bones. One needs to restrict their intake of acidic fruit juices to avoid tooth damage. Coconut water, celery juice and vegetable juice are alkaline and will not harm the teeth.

The data below is from the U.S. FDA Center for Food Safety and Applied Nutrition.

Approximate pH of Foods and Food products

Item	Approximate pH
Apple, eating	3.30 - 4.00
Apricots	3.30 - 4.80
Artichokes, cooked	5.60 - 6.00
Asparagus, cooked	6.03 - 6.16
Avocados	6.27 - 6.58
Bananas	4.50 - 5.20

Bass, sea, broiled	6.58 - 6.78
Blackberries, Washington	3.85 - 4.50
Blueberries, Maine	3.12 - 3.33
Bread, Rye	5.20 - 5.90
Bread, whole wheat	5.47 - 5.85
Broccoli, cooked	6.30 - 6.52
Cabbage	5.20 - 6.80
Cantaloupe	6.13 - 6.58
Carrots	5.88 - 6.40
Cauliflower	5.60
Cauliflower, cooked	6.45 - 6.80
Celery	5.70 - 6.00
Celery, cooked	5.37 - 5.92
Chayote (mirliton), cooked	6.00 - 6.30
Cheese, Cottage	4.75 - 5.02
Cherries, California	4.01 - 4.54
Cherries, Royal Ann	3.80 - 3.83
Cucumbers	5.12 - 5.78
Dates, Dromedary	4.14 - 4.88
Eggplant	5.50 - 6.50
Eggs, new-laid, whole	6.58
Figs, Calamyrna	5.05 - 5.98
Grapes, Concord	2.80 - 3.00
Grapes, Seedless	2.90 - 3.82
Grapefruit	3.00 - 3.75
Grapefruit Juice, canned	2.90 - 3.25
Greens, Mixed, chopped	5.05 - 5.22
Kale, cooked	6.36 - 6.80
Kumquat, Florida	3.64 - 4.25
Lemon Juice	2.00 - 2.60
Lettuce, Boston	5.89 - 6.05
Lettuce, Iceberg	5.70 - 6.13
Lime Juice	2.00 - 2.35
Loquat (if acid pH 3.8)	5.10
Mangoes, ripe	3.40- 4.80
Mangosteen	4.50- 5.00
Melon, Casaba	5.78- 6.00
Melons, Honey dew	6.00 - 6.67
Milk, Sour, fine curd	4.70 - 5.65
Muscadine (Grape)	3.20- 3.40
Nectarines	3.92- 4.18
Olives, green, fermented	3.60 - 4.60
Oranges, Florida	3.69 - 4.34

Orange Juice, California	3.30 - 4.19
Papaya	5.20 - 6.00
Peaches	3.30 - 4.05
Pears, Bartlett	3.50 - 4.60
Persimmons	4.42 - 4.70
Pineapple	3.20 - 4.00
Pineapple Juice, canned	3.30 - 3.60
Plums, Red	3.60 - 4.30
Pomegranate	2.93 - 3.20
Potatoes	5.40 - 5.90
Prunes, dried, stewed	3.63 - 3.92
Raspberries	3.22 - 3.95
Rice, Brown	6.20 - 6.80
Rice, White	6.00 - 6.70
Romaine	5.78 - 6.06
Sauerkraut	3.30 - 3.60
Spinach	5.50 - 6.80
Spinach, cooked	6.60 - 7.18
Squash, acorn, cooked	5.18 - 6.49
Strawberries	3.00 - 3.90
Strawberries, California	3.32 - 3.50
String Beans	5.60
Sweet Potatoes	5.30 - 5.60
Tangerine	3.32 - 4.48
Tomatoes	4.30 - 4.90
Tomatoes, Juice	4.10 - 4.60
Vinegar	2.40 - 3.40
Vinegar, cider	3.10
Watermelon	5.18 - 5.60

RADIOACTIVE CONTAMINATION

Radioactive contamination by medical use is currently much higher than any other man-made source of contamination including bomb testing and nuclear reactors. A leading expert in radiation research confirms this. Dr. John Gofman, a physician who is also a physicist, said his research over the past 10 years supports the U.N.'s conclusion. In 1963 the Atomic Energy Commission asked him to establish a Biomedical Research Division at the Lawrence Livermore National Laboratory to evaluate the health effects of all types of nuclear radiation. By 1969, however, the AEC and the "radiation community" were downplaying his warnings about the risks of radiation. Gofman returned to full-time teaching at Berkeley, switching to emeritus status in 1973.

Below is a chart describing where radiation comes from. Most comes from natural sources like radon gas seeping into houses, while medical x-rays are the greatest source of artificial radiation. Fallout, surprisingly, is only less than .03% of the total. This, of course would change drastically if an all out or even a limited nuclear war occurs.

The problem with nuclear bomb testing fallout is that it accumulates over time in your body, so even though fallout is low now, it has been accumulating for decades in our bodies.

Forty to fifty years ago during the heyday of atmospheric nuclear testing (1962 was the year of the most testing) radioactive fallout was much higher in concentration, especially in the areas near the testing sites.

During the early sixties the country of Ecuador was determined to be the place with the least fallout in the world, due to its high mountains which screen out radioactive fallout.

Radiation Exposure
Natural:
Radon 55%
Cosmic 8%
Terrestrial 8%
Internal 11%
Total Natural 82%

Artificial:
Medical X ray 11%
Nuclear medicine 4%
Consumer products 3%
Other Occupational <0.3
Nuclear Fuel Cycle <0.03
Fallout <0.03 % of total or less than 1 millirem per person
Miscellaneous <0.03
Total Artificial 18%
Total Artificial and Natural 100%
Chart developed by the National Council on Radiation Protection and Measurement (NCRP 93)

THE TRUTH ABOUT
LOW-LEVEL RADIOACTIVE FALLOUT

The book Secret Fallout, Low-Level Radiation from Hiroshima to Three Mile Island by Ernest J. Sternglass (1972), published by McGraw-Hill Book Company is highly recommended to understand the dangers of nuclear radiation. Permission to distribute this book is freely given so long as no modification of the text is made.

From the foreword of the 1981 edition: "WHEN I UNDERTOOK to write the first edition of this book, originally published in 1972 under the title Low-Level Radiation, my primary concern was with the health effects of worldwide fallout from nuclear weapons, particularly on the developing infant in the mother's womb. At that time I also discussed the first evidence for possible health effects of routine releases of radioactivity from nuclear reactors in their ordinary day-to-day operation. In the ten years that have intervened since then, my concerns about the safety of nuclear plants have unfortunately been reinforced far more than I could have anticipated. Not only in the accident at Three Mile Island, whose likely effects on human health are discussed in the present book, but also in the normal operations of many other nuclear plants, there is now growing evidence for rising infant mortality and damage to the newborn. In the decade that has passed, cancer rates increased most sharply in areas closest to the nuclear reactors whose radioactive gas releases were found to rise most strongly, following the earlier pattern of death rates among the newborn described in the original book.

The first fourteen chapters have been left nearly unchanged, while the rest of the present book brings the story up to the present time. It deals with the newly disclosed evidence that the possibility of serious health damage from weapons testing was long known to our government. It also presents the evidence for widespread damage to the learning abilities of the children born in areas of heavy fallout during the period of massive nuclear weapons testing.

What emerges is that in order for major governments to be able to continue threatening the use of their ever-growing stockpiles of weapons to fight and win nuclear wars rather than merely to deter them, they must keep from their own people the severity of the biological damage already done to their children by past nuclear testing and the releases from nuclear reactors near their homes. It is to focus attention on the need to end this hidden threat to the future of human life on this globe that this new edition has been prepared. Ernest J. Sternglass Pittsburgh July 1980."

The following is another important excerpt from the book:
"But the main reason why it seemed that fallout was at least as effective as X-rays in producing childhood cancer was the growing evidence for a direct relationship between the number of X-ray pictures taken and the risk of cancer. For if the risk increased with each additional picture, as the studies of Stewart and MacMahon indicated it did, then this clearly implied that there was no significant healing of the damage and thus that the cancer-causing effects of radiation were cumulative.

All of this evidence combined pointed toward a single tragic conclusion: **Man, especially during the stage of early embryonic life, was hundreds or thousands of times more sensitive to radiation than anyone had ever suspected.**

Apparently it had been decided by the government's scientific advisory groups that it was not necessary to take into account the long-range after-effects of radiation, either on the survivors themselves or on their offspring. Yet, as I well knew from my own research, the reason why so much effort was being spent to reduce the dose from medical X-rays was that the doses of only a few rads per year received by radiologists in the course of their work had been found to decrease their life spans significantly, while among their children there had been a definite increase in congenital defects."

The half-life of Strontium 90 is 28 years. 10 half-lives are needed for an isotope to fully decay, so 280 years are needed to return to normal. The most nuclear bomb testing was in 1962 which is 51 years ago (as of 2013), so we will still get strontium 90 raining down on us for another 229 years. A half-life is the time required for the radioactivity of material taken in by a living organism to be reduced to half its initial value by a combination of biological elimination processes and radioactive decay.

Fallout has been increasing the amount of cancers worldwide. One in four who die, die of cancer in the USA. Of the some 1,372,000 cases of cancer in 2005, about half died. The idea that a nuclear war can be survived is not valid based on the evidence that fallout kills slowly over time. A nuclear winter or mini ice age would occur if a major nuclear war broke out, due to the intensity of smoke and dust being thrown into the atmosphere, clouding the sun.

THE FUKUSHIMA NUCLEAR DISASTER AND FOODS THAT PROTECT AGAINST RADIATION

Dr. Chris Busby, well known world radiation expert, tells us that with his sophisticated equipment, there were areas in Tokyo that were 1000 times higher in radiation, than the exclusion zone (evacuation zone) in Chernobyl.

The distance of Tokyo (35 million people) to Fukushima is only 238.34 kilometers (km) or 148 miles (about the distance of Big Sur, California to San Francisco, California). Northern pacific fish, seafood and seaweed will become contaminated.

The report also said radiation damage from Fukushima was at least 15,000 terrabecquerels (a TBq is 10 to the 12th power) of Cesium 137. For perspective, that is significant as compared to 89 terrabecquerels released by the US uranium bombs in Hiroshima. Chernobyl released 85 petabecquerels (a PBq is 10 to the 15th power) or 85,000 terrabecquerels of Cesium 137 over a longer time period.

Fukushima is predicted to be worse than Chernobyl because Chernobyl only involved 200 tons of fuel whereas Fukushima has about 2,000 tons of reactor fuel and spent fuel which if left alone could get hotter and hotter and vaporize all the radioactive material.

People are predicting that in a year or two all of Northern Japan, which includes Tokyo could become uninhabitable. In a cover up response to this situation, the Japanese government raised exposure level for adults and children from one millisieverts to 20 millisieverts. Twenty millisieverts matches maximum allowable exposure for nuclear industry workers.

Atmospheric nuclear testing, which ended on October 10, 1963 (except for France and China), released something on order of 740 PBq of Cs-137 according to http://www.davistownmuseum.org/cbm/Rad8.html. Chernobyl released 85 PBq or just over one-tenth of what was released during nuclear testing. 15,000 terrabecquerels or 15 PBq of Cesium 137 have been released so far at Fukushima but this figure will climb over time and because there is 10 times more radioactive material at Fukushima than was at Chernobyl.

In Chernobyl spirulina was used to help save many children from radiation poisoning. By taking 5 grams of spirulina a day for 45 days, the Institute of Radiation Medicine in Minsk proved that children on this protocol experienced enhanced immune systems, T-cell counts and reduced radioactivity. Chlorella algae, a known immune system builder and heavy metal detoxifier, has also shown radioprotective effects. Because they bind heavy metals, algae should therefore be consumed after exposure to any type of radioactive contamination.

In 1968 a group of Canadian researchers at McGill University of Montreal, headed by Dr. Stanley Skoryna began researching a method to counteract the effects of nuclear fallout. They found that sodium alginate from kelp reduced radioactive strontium absorption in the intestines by 50 to 80 percent.

The Atomic Energy Commission recommends for maximum protection against radioactive poisoning for humans, taking a minimum of 2 to 3 ounces of sea vegetables a week or 10 grams (two tablespoons) a day of sodium alginate supplements. During or after exposure to radiation, the dosage should be increased to two full tablespoons of sodium alginate four times daily to insure that there is a continual supply in the GI or gastrointestinal tract. There may be a rare concern of constipation but this can be avoided if the sodium alginate is made into a fruit gelatin.

Agar, derived from sodium alginate in kelp, is a safe, nontoxic substance that can be used as a thickening agent or gelatin. Protective foods are: sodium alginate powder, potassium iodide tablets, spirulina, chlorella and the algaes (kelp, dulse etc.), Brassica and high beta carotene vegetables and potassium.

The company Maine Coast Sea Vegetables has sea vegetables that are radiation free. They used University of Maine scientists to test for radioactivity in both fresh and dried samples following the Fukushima disaster. To date, all samples have shown no indication of radioactivity above natural, background levels. They are developing an ongoing testing program for the months and possibly years to come.

THE WORLD WIDE CLIMATE CRISIS

The world wide climate crisis has been accepted as fact by most scientists internationally. The scientific consensus is clearly expressed in the reports of the Intergovernmental Panel on Climate Change (IPCC), created in 1988 by the World Meteorological Organization and the United Nations Environmental Programme. Other major scientific organizations in agreement include the National Academy of Sciences, The American Meteorological Society, the American Geophysical Union and the American Association for the Advancement of Science. The United States military command at the Pentagon is preparing for a crisis situation as the climate destabilizes and causes widespread crop failure and famine.

Despite this general consensus there are a few people that think there is no cause for alarm. They believe that the sun is the natural cause of climate change and not man. One fact that can't be disputed is that man has cut trees to create his artificial, civilized way of life clearing forests to raise grains and to raise animals for meat.

Humans also use the wood cut from forests for buildings, paper and furniture. Deforestation causes desertification as has happened in the northern Sahara desert which was once the fertile breadbasket of Rome. Cutting of forests and then grazing animals on the land creates deserts where temperatures are extremely high and little rain falls. Forests create cloud formation which brings rain and the cooling of the land. Forests provide shade which cools the soil allowing many plants and animals to flourish.

The sun has a part to play in climate change, but so does man. We need to stop all cutting of original growth and regenerating forest because the forests are the lungs of the world, converting carbon dioxide into oxygen.

Carbon dioxide is a dense, heavy gas that traps heat from the sun in a greenhouse like manner by forming a layer in the atmosphere. Carbon dioxide emissions from vehicles, power plants, cities and industries must also be reduced to counter the loss of forest photosynthetic conversion of carbon dioxide into oxygen and to stop air pollution which is destroying the health of those living in and near big cities. Forests need to be replanted in epic proportions. Fruit trees can provide food beside converting CO_2 to oxygen. Evergreen fir trees produce oxygen and negative ions, create homes for animals and produce wood. Pulverized rock re-mineralizes depleted soils insuring healthy growth and disease resistance in natural forested areas and also in planted forests.

A change to a meatless lacto-vegetarian diet or even a semi-lacto-vegetarian (half-time vegetarian) will help stabilize the climate, since meat is the number one culprit in the climate crisis. According to Mongabay.com, a source used by CNN, CBS, the Discovery Channel, NBC, UPI, Yahoo and several other outlets, "Cattle ranching is the leading cause of deforestation in the Brazilian Amazon. This has been the case since at least the 1970s: government figures attributed 38% of deforestation from 1966-1975 to large scale cattle ranching. However, today the situation may be even worse. According to The Center for International Forestry Research (CIFOR), "Between 1990 and 2001 the percentage of Europe's processed meat imports that came from Brazil rose from 40 to 74 percent" and by 2003 "For the first time ever, the growth in Brazilian cattle production-80 percent of which was in the Amazon-was largely export driven."

References

Baibas N, Trichopoulou A, Voridis E, & Trichopoulos D. (2005). Residence in mountainous compared with lowland areas in relation to total and coronary mortality. A study in rural Greece. *Journal of Epidemiology and Community Health, 59*(4), 274–278

Batchelor, A. J. et al. (1983). Reduced plasma half-life of radio-labeled 25-hydroxy vitamin D3 in subjects receiving a high-fiber diet. *British Journal of Nutrition, 49*, 213-216.

Ben-Arye E., Goldin E., Wengrower D., Stamper A., Kohn R., & Berry E. (2002). Wheat grass juice in the treatment of active distal ulcerative colitis: a randomized double-blind placebo-controlled trial. *Scandinavian Journal Gastroenterology, 37*(4), 444-9.

Bent, S., Kane, C., Shinohara, K., et al. (2006). Saw palmetto for benign prostatic hyperplasia. *New England Journal of Medicine, 354*(6), 557-566.

Blankenhorn, D. H., Johnson, R. L., Mack, W. J., el Zein, H. A., & Vailas, L. I. (1990). The influence of diet on the appearance of new lesions in human coronary arteries. *JAMA, 263*(12), 1646-52.

Bonthuis, M., Hughes, M. C., Ibiebele, T. I., Green, A. C., & van der Pols, J. C. (2010). Dairy consumption and patterns of mortality of Australian adults. *European Journal Clinical Nutrition, 64*(6), 569-77.

Briley, M., Carilla, E., & Roger, A. (1984). Inhibitory effect of permixon on testosterone 5a-reductase activity of the rat ventral prostate. *British Journal of Pharmacology, 83*(suppl.), 401P.

Burr, G. O., & Burr, M. M. (1929). A new deficiency disease produced by the rigid exclusion of fat from the diet. *Journal of Biological Chemistry, 82*, 345-367.

Burr, G. O., & Burr, M. M. (1930). On the nature and role of the fatty acids essential in nutrition. *Journal of Biological Chemistry, 86*, 587-621

Burr, M. L., Ashfield-Watt, P. A., Dunstan, F. D., Fehily, A. M., Breay, P., Ashton, T., Zotos, P. C., Haboubi, N. A., & Elwood, P. C. (2003). Lack of benefit of dietary advice to men with angina: results of a controlled trial. *European Journal of Clinical Nutrition, 57*(2), 193-200.

Campbell, T. C., Campbell, II T. M., & Carpenter, K. (2003). The china study. A short history of nutritional science: Part 2, (1885-1912). *Journal of Nutrition, 133*(4), 975-84.

Carraro, J. C., Raynaud, J. P., Koch, G., Chisholm, G. D., Di Silverio, F., Teillac P., et al. (1996). Comparison of phytotherapy (permixon) with finasteride in the treatment of benign prostate hyperplasia: a randomized international study of 1,098 patients. *Prostate, 29*, 231–40.

Casadesus, G., Shukitt-Hale, B., Stellwagen, H. M., et al. (2004). Modulation of hippocampal plasticity and cognitive behavior by short-term blueberry supplementation in aged rats. *Nutritional Neuroscience, 7*(5-6), 309-16.

Clement, M. R., et al. (1987). A new mechanism for induced vitamin D deficiency in calcium deprivation. *Nature, 325*, 62-65.

Cordain, L. (1999). Cereal grains: Humanity's double-edged sword. *World Review of Nutrition and Dietetics, 84*, 19-73.

Dagnelie, P. C., et al. (1990) High prevalence of rickets in infants on macrobiotic diets. *American Journal Clinical Nutrition, 51*, 202-208.

Di Silverio, F., D'Eramo, G., Lubrano, C., Flammia, G. P., Sciarra, A., Palma, E., et al. (1992). Evidence that serenoa repens extract displays an anti-estrogenic activity in prostatic tissue of benign prostatic hypertrophy patients. *European Urology, 21*, 309-14.

Elwood, P. C., Pickering, J. E., Hughes, J., Fehily, A. M., & Ness, A. R. (2004). Milk drinking, ischaemic heart disease and ischaemic stroke II. evidence from cohort studies. *European Journal of Clinical Nutrition, 58*(5), 718-24.

Elwood, P. C., Strain, J. J., Robson, P. J., Fehily, A. M., Hughes, J., Pickering, J., & Ness A. (2005). Milk consumption, stroke, and heart attack risk: evidence from the Caerphilly cohort of older men. *Journal of Epidemiology and Community Health, 59*(6), 502-5.

Epel E. S., Blackburn E. H., Lin J., Dhabhar F. S., Adler N. E., Morrow J. D., & Cawthon R. M. (2004). Accelerated telomere shortening in response to life stress. *Proceedings National Academy of Science, 101*(49), 17312-5.

Felton, C. V., Crook, D., Davies, M. J., & Oliver, M. F. (1994). Dietary polyunsaturated fatty acids and composition of human aortic plaques. *Lancet, 344*(8931), 1195-6.

Fraser, G., et al. (1991). Diet and lung cancer in seventh day adventists. *American Journal of Epidemiology, 133,* 683-93.

Fraser, L. (2000, February 4). The French Paradox. Salon. Retrieved January 31, 2012, from http://www.salon.com/2000/02/04/paradox

Fu, M. X., Requena, J. R., Jenkins, A. J., Lyons, T. J., Baynes, J. W., & Thorpe, S. R. (1996). The advanced glycation end product, nepsilon-(carboxymethyl)lysine, is a product of both lipid peroxidation and glycoxidation reactions. *Journal of Biological Chemistry, 271*(17), 9982-6.

Geleijnse, J. M., Vermeer, C., Grobbee, D. E., Schurgers, L. J., Knapen, M. H., van der Meer, I. M., Hofman, A., & Witteman, J. C. (2004). Dietary intake of menaquinone is associated with a reduced risk of coronary heart disease: the rotterdam study. *Journal of Nutrition, 134*(11), 3100-5.

Gerber, G. S., Kuznetsov, D., Johnson, B. C., & Burstein, J. D. (2001). Randomized, double-blind, placebo-controlled trial of saw palmetto in men with lower urinary tract symptoms. *Urology, 58,* 960–4.

Golub, M. S., et al. (1996). Adolescent growth and maturation in zinc-deprived rhesus monkeys. *American Journal of Clinical Nutrition, 64,* 274-282.

Grant, et al. (1982). The effect of heating on the haemagglutinating activity and nutritional properties of bean *(Phaseolus vulgaris) seeds. Journal of the Science of Food and Agriculture, 33,* 324-1326.

Gupta, Y. P. (1987). Anti-nutritional and toxic factors in food legumes A review. *Plant Foods for Human Nutrition, 37,* 201-228.

Guyton, A. C. (1996). *Textbook of medical physiology.* Philadelphia, PA: W.B. Saunders Company.

Hänninen O, Rauma AL, Kaartinen K, & Nenonen M. (1999). Vegan diet in physiological health promotion. *Acta Physiologica Academiae Scientiarum Hungaricae, 86*(3-4), 171-80.

Harris, R. C., Tallon, M. J., Dunnett, M., Boobis, L., Coakley, J., Kim, H. J., Fallowfield, J. L., Hill, C. A., Sale, C., & Wise, J. A. (2006). The absorption of orally supplied beta-alanine and its effect on muscle carnosine synthesis in human vastus lateralis. *Amino Acids, 30*(3), 279-89.

Hass, E. M. (1995). *Staying healthy with nutrition: The complete guide to diet and nutritional medicine.* Berkeley, CA: Celestial Arts.

Hauck, D. W. (1998). Alchemical Properties of Foods Retrieved November 10, 2008, from http://www.alchemylab.com/guideto.htm

Hauswirth, C. B., Scheeder M. R., & Beer, J. H. (2004). High omega-3 fatty acid content in alpine cheese: the basis for an alpine paradox. *Circulation, 109*(1), 103-7.

He, F. J., MacGregor, G. A. (2009). A comprehensive review on salt and health and current experience of worldwide salt reduction programmes. *Journal of Human Hypertension,* (6), 363-84.

Hermansen, K., Rasmussen O, Gregersen, S., & Larsen, S. (1992). Influence of ripeness of banana on the blood glucose and insulin response in type 2 diabetic subjects. *Diabetic Medicine, 9,* 730-43.

Hill, C. A., Harris, R. C., Kim, H. J., Harris, B. D., Sale, C., Boobis, L. H., Kim, C. K., & Wise, J. A. (2007). Influence of beta-alanine supplementation on skeletal muscle carnosine concentrations and high intensity cycling capacity. *Amino Acids, 32*(2), 225-33.

Howell, E. (1985). *Enzyme nutrition.* Avery Publishing, Wayne, New Jersey.

Karppanen, H., & Mervaala, E. (2006). Sodium intake and hypertension. *Progress in Cardiovascular Diseases, 49*(2), 59-75

Kramer, Martha M., Latzke, F., & Shaw, M. M. (1928). A comparison of raw, pasteurized, evaporated and dried milks as sources of calcium and phosphorus for the human subject. *Journal of Biological Chemistry, 79,* 283-295.

Kripke, D. F., Garfinkel, L., Wingard D. L., Klauber, M. R., & Marler, M. R. (2002). Mortality associated with sleep duration and insomnia. *Archives of General Psychiatry, 59,* 131-136.

Lau, F. C., Shukitt-Hale, B., & Joseph, J. A. (2005) The beneficial effects of fruit polyphenols on brain aging. *Neurobiology of Aging, 26S,* S128-S132.

Leitzmann, M. F. et al. (2004). Dietary intake of n–3 and n–6 fatty acids and the risk of prostate cancer. *American Journal of Clinical Nutrition, 80*(1), 204-216.

Liener, I. E. (1994). Implications of anti-nutritional components in soybean foods. *Critical Reviews in Food Science and Nutrition, 34,* 31-67.

Lindeberg, S., & Lundh, B. (1993). Apparent absence of stroke and ischaemic heart disease in a traditional melanesian island: a clinical study in kitava. *Journal of Internal Medicine, 233*(3), 269-75.

Liu, J., Atamna, H., Kuratsune, H., & Ames, B. N. (2002). Delaying brain mitochondrial decay and aging with mitochondrial antioxidants and metabolites. *Annals NY Academy of Science, 959,* 133-66.

Lowe, F. C., & Ku, J. C. (1996). Phytotherapy in treatment of benign prostatic hyperplasia: A critical review. *Urology, 48,* 12–20.

Luevano-Contreras, C., & Chapman-Novakofski, K. (2010). Dietary advanced glycation end products and aging. *Nutrients, 2*(12), 1247–1265.

Marawaha R. K., Bansal D., Kaur, S., & Trehan, A. (2004). Effect of wheat grass therapy on transfusion requirement in beta-thalassemia major. *Indian Pediatrics, 41*(7), 716-20.

Marks, L. S., Hess, D. L., Dorey, F. J., Macairan, M. L., Cruz Santos, P. B., & Tyler, V. E. (2001) Tissue effects of saw palmetto and finasteride: Use of biopsy cores for in situ quantification of prostatic androgens. *Urology, 57,* 999–1005.

Marks, L. S., Partin, A. W., Epstein, J. I., Tyler, V. E., Simon, I., Macairan, M. L., et al. (2000). Effects of a saw palmetto herbal blend in men with symptomatic benign prostatic hyperplasia. *Journal of Urology, 163,* 1451–6.

Matchett, M. D., Mackinnon, S. L., Sweeney, M. I., Gottschall-Pass, K. T., & Hurta, R. A. (2005). Blueberry flavonoids inhibit matrix metalloproteinase activity in DU145 human prostate cancer cells. *Biochemistry and Cell Biology, 83*(5), 637-43.

McPherson J. D., Shilton B. H., & Walton D. J., (1988). Role of fructose in glycation and cross-linking of proteins. *Biochemistry, 22,27*(6), 1901-7.

Merriam Webster Dictionary online. (2008). Retrieved November 10, 2008 from http://www.merriam-webster.com/dictionary/transition

Mori, A., Lehmann, S., O'Kelly, J., Kumagai, T., Desmond, J. C., Pervan, M., McBride, W. H., Kizaki, M., & Koeffler, H. P. (2006). Capsaicin, a component of red peppers, inhibits the growth of androgen-independent, p53 mutant prostate cancer cells. *Cancer Research, 66*(6), 3222-9.

Pan, A., Sun, Q., Bernstein, A. M., Schulze, M. B., Manson, J. E., Stampfer, M. J., Willett, W. C., & Hu, F. B. (2012). Red meat consumption and mortality: results from 2 prospective cohort studies. *Archives of Internal Medicine. 172*(7), 555-63.

Plosker, G. L., & Brogden, R. N. (1996). Serenoa repens (permixon). A review of its pharmacology and therapeutic efficacy in benign prostatic hyperplasia. *Drugs and Aging, 9,* 379–95.

Preston J. E., Hipkiss A. R., Himsworth D.T., Romero IA, & Abbott J. N. (1998). Toxic effects of beta-amyloid(25-35) on immortalised rat brain endothelial cell: protection by carnosine, homocarnosine and beta-alanine. *Neuroscience Letters, 242*(2), 105-8.

Price, Weston A. (2008). *Nutrition and physical degeneration.* Lemon Grove, CA: Price Pottenger Nutrition.

Prokop, O. (1990). The herbst-volkheimer effect. (Article in German). *Kitasato Archives of Experimental Medicine, 63*(1), 1-6.

Puterman, E., Lin, J., Blackburn, E., O'Donovan, A., Adler, N., & Epel, E. (2010). The power of exercise: buffering the effect of chronic stress on telomere length. *Public Library of Science, One, 5*(5), e10837.

Robinson, W. (1948). Delay in the appearance of palpable mammary tumors in C3H mice following the ingestion of pollenized food. Journal of the National Cancer Institute, 9(2), 119-23. Singh, P. & Fraser, G. (1998). Dietary risk factors for colon cancer in a low-risk population.

American Journal of Epidemiology, 148(8), 761-774.

Schneider, H., Steenbock, H., & Platz, B. R. (1940). Essential fatty acids, vitamin B6, and other factors in the cure of rat acrodynia. *Journal of Biological Chemistry 132*, 539-551.

Small, J. K., Bombardelli, E, & Morazzoni, P. (1997). Serenoa repens (bartram). *Fitoterapia, 68*, 99–113.

Staessen, J. et al. (2011). Fatal and nonfatal outcomes, incidence of hypertension, and blood pressure changes in relation to urinary sodium excretion. *Journal of the American Medical Association, 305*, 1777 - 1785.

Stokes, K. A., Nevill, M. E., Hall, G. M., & Lakomy, H. K. (2002). The time course of the human growth hormone response to a 6 s and a 30 s cycle ergometer sprint. *Journal of Sports Sciences, (6)*, 487-94.

Veierød, M.B., Thelle, D.S., & Laake, P. (1997). Diet and risk of cutaneous malignant melanoma: a prospective study of 50,757 norwegian men and women. *International Journal of Cancer. 71*(4), 600-4.

Warensjö, E., Jansson, J. H., Cederholm, T., Boman, K., Eliasson, M., Hallmans, G., Johansson, I., & Sjögren, P. (2010). Biomarkers of milk fat and the risk of myocardial infarction in men and women: a prospective, matched case-control study. *American Journal of Clinical Nutrition, 92*(1), 194-202.

Watson, George. (1972). Nutrition and Your Mind: The psychochemical response. New York: HarperCollins.

West, C. Samuel (1981). *The golden seven plus one.* Orem, Utah: Samuel Publishing Company.

Willetts, K. E., Clements, M. S., Champion, S., et al. (2003). Serenoa repens extract for benign prostate hyperplasia: A randomized controlled trial. *British Journal of Urology International, 92*(3), 267-270.

Wilt, T., Ishani, A., & MacDonald, R. (2002). Serenoa repens for benign prostatic hyperplasia. *Cochrane Database of Systematic Reviews, 3*, CD00142.

Worthington, V. (2001). Nutritional quality of organic versus conventional fruits, vegetables, and grains. *The Journal of Alternative and*

Complementary Medicine, 7(2), 161-173.

Xu, Q., Parks, C. G., DeRoo, L. A., Cawthon R. M., Sandler D. P., & Chen, H. (2009). Multivitamin use and telomere length in women. *American Journal of Clinical Nutrition, (6)*, 1857-63.

Zhang, R., Humphreys, I., Sahu, R. P., Shi, Y., & Srivastava, S. K. (2008). In vitro and in vivo induction of apoptosis by capsaicin in pancreatic cancer cells is mediated through ROS generation and mito-chondrial death pathway. *Apoptosis, (12)*, 1465-78.

Suggested Further Reading

The Buddhist Bible. Goddard, Dwight. Boston, USA: Beacon Press, 1938. An excellent collection of Buddhist scriptures.

The Buddhist Essene Gospel of Jesus Vol. I, II & III, Unveiling the Gospel's Divine Mysteries, The New Age Essene and Maha Bodhi Renaissance & The Disciple Whom Jesus Loved, And The Counterfeit Zealot Messianists. Lovewisdom, Johnny. Paradisian publications, 2004, 2007, 2012.

The Cause and Cure of Human Illness. Ehret, Prof. Arnold. The Ehret Literature Publishing Company, Inc. P O Box 24 Dobbs Ferry, New York 10522-0024 www.arnoldehret.org.

Chi Nei Tsang Internal Organs Chi Massage. Chia, Maneewan and Chia, Mantak. Huntington: Healing Tao Books, 1991.

The Colon Health Handbook. Gray, Robert. Reno, USA: Emerald Publishing, 1990.

Enzyme Nutrition. Howell, Edward. New Jersey: Avery Publishing, 1985. The food enzyme bible.

Forest Gardening. Hart, Robert. White River Junction: Chelsea Green Publishing Company, 1996. A good introduction to the idea of a 7 level low maintenance fruit forest.

Golden Path to Rejuvenation. Krok, Morris. South Africa: Essence of Health, 1964.

The Golden Seven Plus One. West, Corwyn Samuel. Orem, Utah, USA: Samuel Publishing Company P.O. Box 1051 Orem, Utah 84057, 1981.

Healing Love Through the Tao: Cultivating Female Sexual Energy. Mantak Chia, Maneewan Chia, Huntington: Healing Tao Books, 1991.

The Holy Science. Sri Yukteswar. Los Angeles, USA: Self-Realization Fellowship, 1990. The Self Realization Fellowship of California 3880 San Rafael Avenue, Los Angeles CA, USA 90065. Many fruitarian references.

How to Grow More Vegetables: And Fruits, Nuts, Berries, Grains, and Other Crops Than You Ever Thought Possible on Less Land Than You Can Imagine. Jeavons, John. Berkeley, CA, USA: Ten Speed Press, 6th edition, 2002.

How to Grow Vegetables and Fruits by the Organic Method. Rodale, J. I. Emmaus: Rodale Press, 1976.

How to Make a Forest Garden. Whitefield, Patrick. Clanfield, Hants: Permanent Publications, 1996. Create a low-maintenance food-producing garden using the ecological principles of a natural woodland.

Introduction to Permaculture. Mollison, Bill. Sisters Creek, Tasmania: Tagari Publications, 1997.

The Mucusless Diet Healing System. Ehret, Prof. Arnold. The Ehret Literature Publishing Company, Inc. P O Box 24 Dobbs Ferry, New York 10522-0024 www.arnoldehret.org.

Noah's Garden: Restoring the Ecology of Our Own Back Yards. Stein, Sara. Boston: Houghton Mifflin, 1993.

Taoist Secrets of Love: Cultivating Male Sexual Energy. Mantak Chia, Michael Winn. Aurora, IL, USA: Aurora Press, 1984.

CPSIA information can be obtained
at www.ICGtesting.com
Printed in the USA
LVOW10s1511150517
534580LV00001B/291/P